Levene's color atlas of
Dermatology
second edition

D1323936

Gary White
MD

Assistant Clinical Professor
University of California
San Diego
California
USA

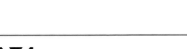
Mosby-Wolfe

London • Baltimore • Barcelona • Bogotá • Boston
Buenos Aires • Carlsbad, CA • Chicago • Madrid
Mexico City • Milan • Naples, FL • New York
Philadelphia • St Louis • Seoul • Singapore
Sydney • Taipei • Tokyo • Toronto • Wiesbaden

To Olivia and Benjamin, my precious children.

Publisher:	**Richard Furn**
Development Editor:	**Jennifer Prast**
Project Manager:	**Sarah Gray**
Index:	**Jill Halliday**
Cover Design:	**Greg Smith**

Copyright © 1997 Times Mirror International Publishers Limited

Published in 1997 by Mosby-Wolfe, an imprint of Times Mirror International Publishers Limited

Printed in Italy by Vincenzo Bona s.r.l., Turin

ISBN 0 7234 2552 3

For full details of all Times Mirror International Publishers Limited titles, please write to Times Mirror International Publishers Limited, Lynton House, 7–12 Tavistock Square, London WC1H 9LB, England.

A CIP catalogue record for this book is available from the British Library.

Contents

Foreword

More than twenty years ago, Peter Wolfe had the brilliant idea of publishing a series of inexpensive, easy-to-handle color atlases on a wide range of subjects, suitable for medical students and junior doctors. The series was an immediate success and soon appeared in other languages, ensuring that the Wolfe Color Atlas gained worldwide recognition.

Two subjects naturally presented themselves as suitable for the Wolfe approach – anatomy and dermatology. The first edition of Levene and Calnan's *Color Atlas of Dermatology* has now sold over 400,000 copies. The demand for a second edition was self-evident. It is tragic that Gerald Levene died so unexpectedly from a heart attack whilst heavily involved in his preparations for it.

The burden was transferred to the willing shoulders of Dr Gary M White at the University of California in San Diego. It was not an easy task. Like most branches of medicine, dermatology has changed over the past two decades. The second edition needed to reflect these changes and yet remain appropriate to the readership. The range of dermatology is now so vast that the choice of what to include or omit must have been extremely difficult. The decisions are those of the author, based on his experience and knowledge of medical students and junior doctors.

A second edition after twenty years had to be different to reflect progress and change; Dr White has not evaded his responsibilities in this regard. Gerald Levene would be as gratified as I am by the result. It is a fitting memorial to Levene's endeavours and achievements over so many years.

Charles D Calnan

Section 1

Morphology

Morphology

MORPHOLOGIC AND DESCRIPTIVE TERMINOLOGY

The importance of using the correct terms when describing a dermatologic condition cannot be over-emphasized. To the uninitiated, every rash is 'maculopapular'. The majority of dermatologic diseases, however, are not. In addition to its morphology, a lesion's color, number, configuration and distribution are of vital importance. Much of the process of learning dermatology involves learning its language. The following pages contain illustrations of some of these terms.

MORPHOLOGIC TERMS (see pages 4–7)

Macule/patch A color change of the skin only. There is no elevation, induration or scale. If you close your eyes and feel only, you can not tell it is there. The difference between a macule and a patch is one of size, i.e. a patch is greater than 1 cm in diameter.

Papule/nodule A raised spot on the surface of skin. The difference between a papule and a nodule is one of size, i.e. a nodule is greater than 5 mm. The word tumor is sometimes used to describe a large nodule (see **Figure ii**).

Plaque A raised uniform thickening of a portion of the skin with a well-defined edge and a flat or rough surface (see **Figure iii**).

Vesicle/bulla A fluid-filled blister. The term vesicle is used if the lesion is less than 5 mm, and the term bulla is used if the lesion is greater than 5 mm (see **Figure iv**).

Pustule A bleb of skin filled with pus.

Fissure A crack or split in the epidermis (see **Figure v**).

Erosion An area of partial loss of the epidermis (see **Figure vi**).

Ulcer An area of total loss of the epidermis (see **Figure vii**).

Atrophy/lipoatrophy   Atrophy is loss of thickness or substance of the epidermis or dermis. Lipoatrophy is loss of the subcutaneous fat.

Wheal   A transient pink plaque caused by edema of the skin, usually restricted to describing urticaria.

Petechia/purpura   Purple discoloration of the skin caused by the extravasation of blood. A lesion less than 5 mm is a petechia, one greater than 5 mm is called purpura.

Papulosquamous   This term is used to describe conditions that manifest themselves as papules or plaques with scale, e.g. psoriasis, lichen planus, pityriasis rubra pilaris.

Eczematous   This term is used to describe inflammatory conditions of the skin that appear erythematous and scaly with ill-defined borders, e.g. atopic dermatitis, irritant dermatitis, tinea, etc.

Necrosis   Death of the skin.

SURFACE CHANGES (see pages 7–8)

Scaly   Covered by flakes of flat horny cells loosened from the horny layer (i.e. the stratum corneum) (see **Figure viii**).

Wet/oozing   The water barrier of the skin has been damaged and there is enough flow of fluid from below to keep the surface of the lesion wet.

Crusted   Usually refers to dried serum, but sometimes the term is applied to a thick mass of horny cells or to a mixture of both (see **Figure ix**).

Excoriated   This term means that the lesion has been scratched. The presence of linear erosions or scabs indicates this fact. Old excoriations may turn into linear white scars.

Lichenified   Thickening of the epidermis with an exaggeration of normal skin lines (see **Figure x**).

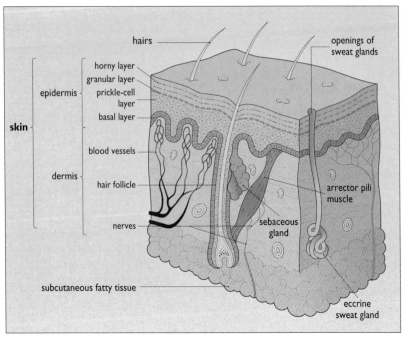

Figure i.
Diagram of skin structure

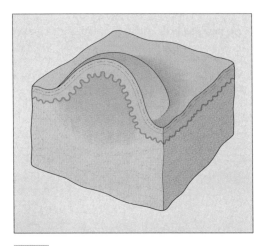

Figure ii.
Papule/nodule

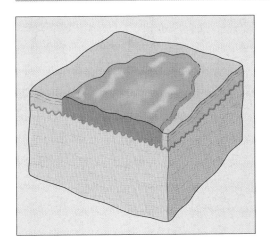

Figure iii.
Plaque

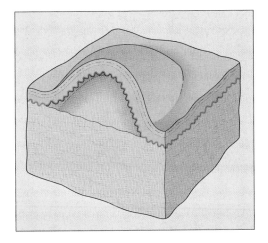

Figure iv.
Vesicle/bulla

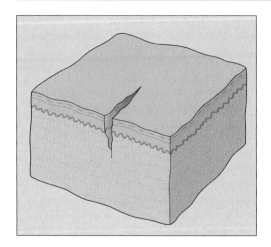

Figure v.
Fissure

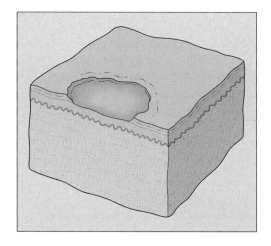

Figure vi.
Erosion

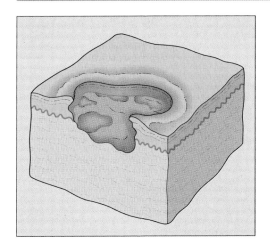

Figure vii.
Ulcer

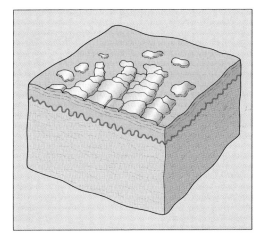

Figure viii.
Scaly

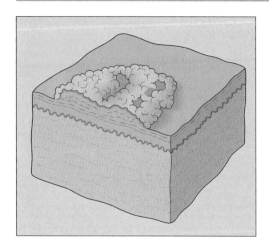

Figure ix.
Crusted

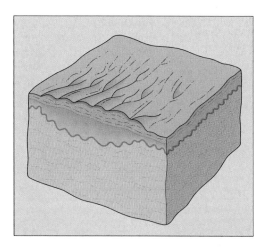

Figure x.
Lichenified

Section 2

Pediatric Dermatology

Congenital and Newborn Diseases

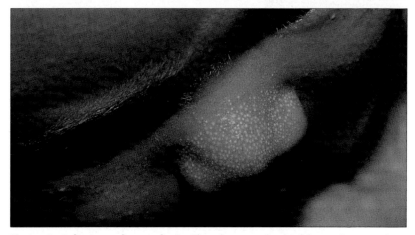

Figure 1. Sebaceous hyperplasia. The sebaceous glands of the newborn may be temporarily enlarged at birth secondary to stimulation by maternal hormones. Note the pinpoint yellow papules on this infant's nose.

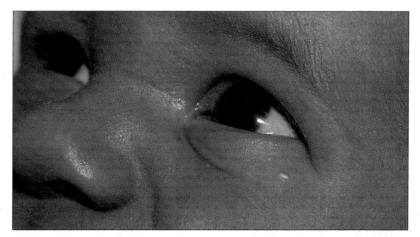

Figure 2. Milia. Small, white milia are common on the face of newborns. Spontaneous resolution is expected.

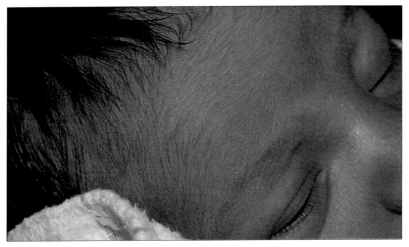

Figure 3. Lanugo hair. The presence of increased hair in an infant, as shown here on the forehead, is common and temporary.

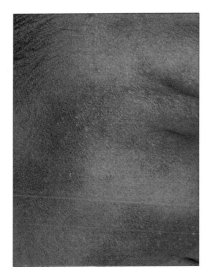

Figure 4. Erythema toxicum.
Erythematous patches, 1–3 cm in diameter, with a central papulopustule in a newborn are characteristic of this benign and transient condition.

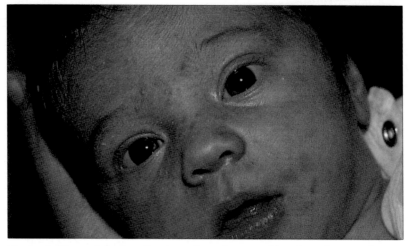

Figure 5. Neonatal acne. Papules and pustules on the face of an infant, usually in the first month of life, are characteristic. Spontaneous resolution occurs.

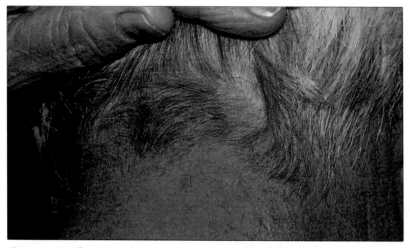

Figure 6. Erythema nuchae. A congenital vascular patch on the nape occurs very commonly and may persist throughout life.

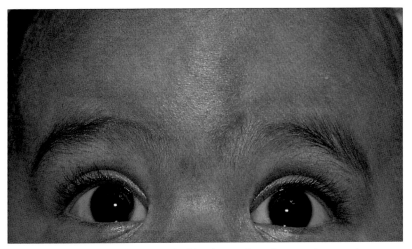

Figure 7. Salmon patch. A vascular blanching red patch or streak across the forehead and/or glabella occurs in many newborn infants. It usually fades, in contrast to port wine stains or vascular patches on the nape, which persist.

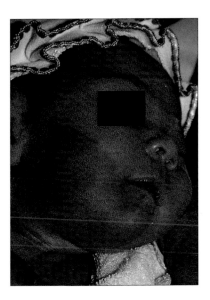

Figure 8. Port wine stain. A congenital, fixed, flat, red or pink patch is characteristic of a port wine stain. The distribution often follows a dermatome, which influences management. Facial port wine stains involving V1 may be associated with ocular abnormalities (e.g. glaucoma, choroidal angioma) with or without Sturge–Weber syndrome. The child shown here with a port wine stain of V3 is at risk for neither. Cosmesis is the main concern.

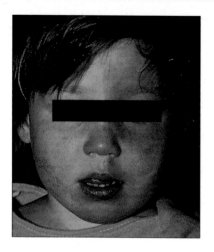

Figure 9. Sturge–Weber syndrome.
A non-inherited disorder that combines a facial port wine stain involving the V1 dermatome (forehead, upper and lower eyelid, and side of the nose), seizures, and ipsilateral leptomeningial angiomatosis. If the port wine stain is in the V2 (upper lip, cheek) or V3 (lower lip, chin, jawline, ear and preauricular) dermatome without involvement of V1, there is no need to rule out Sturge–Weber syndrome. Involvement of V1, V2 and V3, as shown here, significantly increases the risk of Sturge–Weber syndrome.

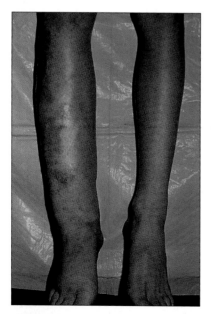

Figure 10. Klippel–Trenaunay syndrome. A congenital nevus flammeus (also known as port wine stain) along with ipsilateral hypertrophy of the bones and/or soft tissue occur together in this syndrome. An extremity is usually affected. Varicose veins develop later in the majority and can cause pain and swelling. (Courtesy of Michael O Murphy, MD.)

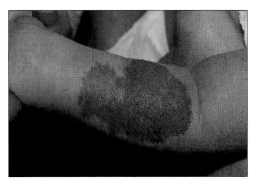

Figure 11. Capillary hemangioma. Capillary hemangiomas are more common in preterm infants and females (female to male ratio of 3:1). At birth they may present as a barely visible, white, anemic stain; a faint, telangiectatic lesion; a flat, red patch, as shown here; a blue spot mimicking a bruise; or rarely a full grown hemangioma.

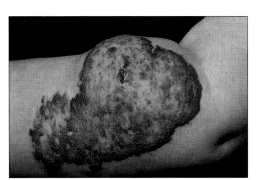

Figure 12. Capillary hemangioma. Capillary hemangiomas are distinguished from vascular malformations (e.g. port wine stain, arteriovenous malformation) by the fact that they proliferate, typically during the first 3–9 months of life. The picture shows the same child shown in **Figure 11** several weeks later.

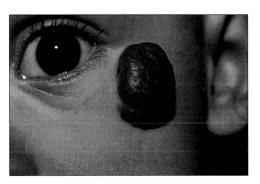

Figure 13. Capillary hemangioma, periocular. If this hemangioma were to grow to the point that it obstructed vision, treatment would be mandatory. Otherwise, permanent visual impairment could result.

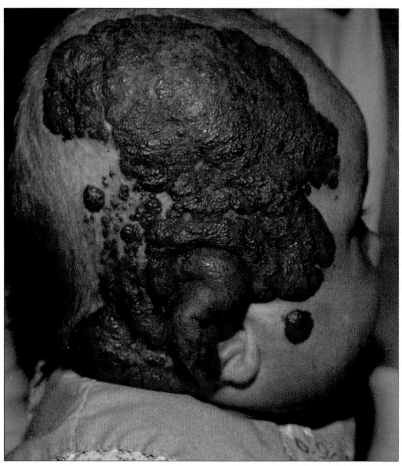

Figure 14. Capillary hemangioma, large. Occasionally, hemangiomas may become rather large and disfiguring. Potential complications include ulceration, bleeding, infection, high output cardiac failure and Kasabach–Merritt syndrome. Large facial hemangiomas may be associated with brain malformations, e.g. the Dandy–Walker malformation. Hemangiomas overlying the anterior neck may be associated with airway involvement and obstruction. (Courtesy of Michael O Murphy, MD.)

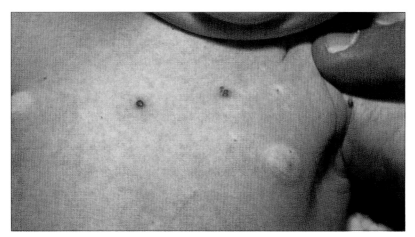

Figure 15. Capillary hemangioma, multiple. Multiple, small hemangiomas occasionally occur and are usually unassociated with internal involvement. Rarely, many large lesions are associated with liver or other systemic hemangiomas. (Courtesy of Michael O Murphy, MD.)

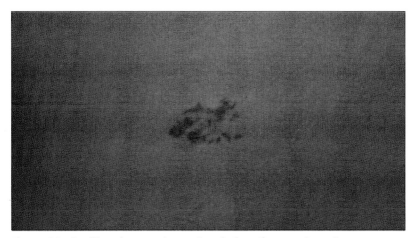

Figure 16. Capillary hemangioma, involuting. If untreated, capillary hemangiomas may spontaneously involute, leaving normal skin, slight redness, telangiectasias, wrinkling and/or sagging. Such spontaneous resolution occurs in 50% of patients by 5 years and 70% by 7 years. The site of a previous hemangioma in this 3-year-old child shows telangiectasias and slight hypopigmentation.

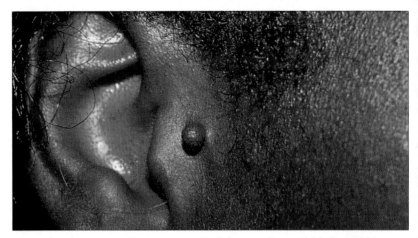

Figure 17. Accessory tragus. A congenital, firm papule or multilobular nodule occurring in the preauricular area is characteristic. The lesion may consist of only skin or skin and cartilage. These lesions may occasionally be bilateral, familial or occur in association with other facial abnormalities.

Figure 18. Accessory nipple. Also known as polythelia, this lesion appears as a small, brown papule which may resemble a nipple, along the milk line that stretches from the axilla through the normal nipple to the groin. One, two (as shown) or more may occur. If two occur, they often appear on opposite sides at the same level. There is an equal sex and side incidence.

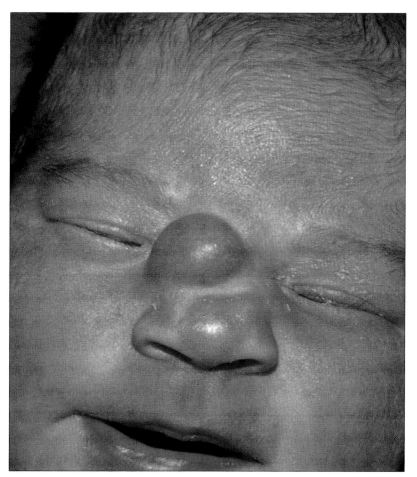

Figure 19. Nasal glioma. The nasal glioma represents a congenital deposit of brain tissue. There is no connection with the central nervous system, in contrast to an encephalocele or meningocele. A congenital, firm, non-transilluminating, blue or red nodule just lateral to the nasal root is characteristic. It does not change size or shape as a result of crying or straining, nor does it distend with jugular vein compression. Imaging of the central nervous system is mandatory prior to biopsy or removal.

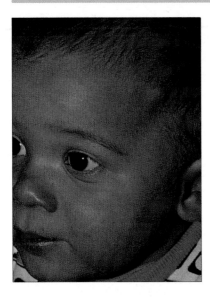

Figure 20. Dermoid cyst. The dermoid cyst results from a sequestration of cutaneous elements along embryonic lines of fusion. A firm or rubbery, painless nodule present congenitally or noticed in the first 2 decades of life is characteristic. It tends to occur on the scalp and face, especially at the lateral third of the eyebrow. An underlying sinus may be present and extend to the scalp, the skull, the extradural space or within the subarachnoid space. This child's dermoid cyst is seen above the temple along the hair line.

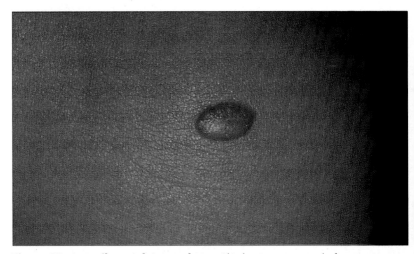

Figure 21. Juvenile xanthogranuloma. This benign tumor results from a proliferation in the skin of histiocytes. A yellowish-red papulonodule in a newborn or young child is characteristic, although adults may be affected. They may be multiple and, rarely, systemic. If untreated, spontaneous resolution usually occurs over months to years.

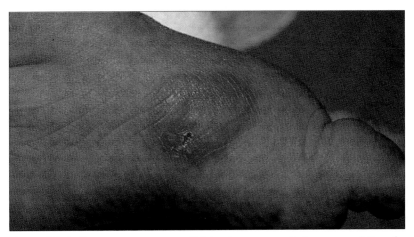

Figure 22. Solitary mastocytoma. This benign tumor results from accumulation of mast cells in the skin. It may be present at birth or develop within the first few weeks of life. It may have an orange-peel surface and will urticate (Darier's sign) or even blister on stroking. Note the reddish-orange color. (See also **Figures 98–100.**)

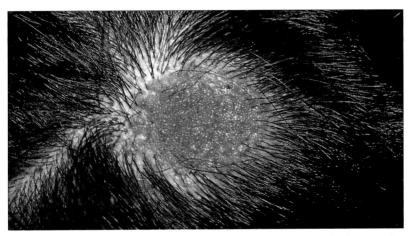

Figure 23. Nevus sebaceous. A round or oval, red to yellow, smooth plaque on the scalp at birth is characteristic. The face is the second most commonly affected site. At puberty, under hormonal influence, the plaque may become verrucous or studded with multiple papules—like a mulberry. Many appendageal neoplasms—both benign and malignant—may develop within the nevus sebaceous. Syringocystadenoma papilliferum or basal cell carcinoma are the most common.

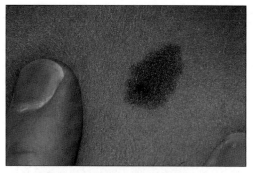

Figure 24. Congenital nevomelanocytic nevus, small. This lesion results from a congenital deposition of nevomelanocytic cells. It usually grows as the patient grows. Melanoma can develop but such an event is rare. Any focal change should be considered for biopsy. The new pigmented spot in this lesion was benign.

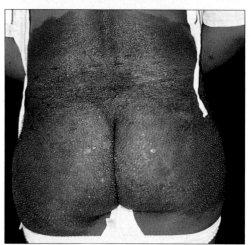

Figure 25. Congenital nevomelanocytic nevus, giant. An extensive, black, verrucous, congenital nevus covering a large area of the body—commonly including the low back and thighs—is characteristic. Multiple smaller, satellite lesions may be scattered over the rest of the skin and even mucous membranes The incidence of developing melanoma is significant, with most estimates between 2 and 6%. (Courtesy of Theodore Sebastian, MD.)

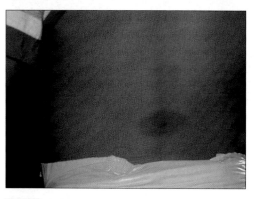

Figure 26. Mongolian spot. A congenital blue-black patch on the sacrum of an Oriental is characteristic. Blacks and less frequently Whites may also be affected. This lesion tends to fade over time. It results from presence of melanin-containing cells within the dermis. The bluish color results from the Tyndall effect.

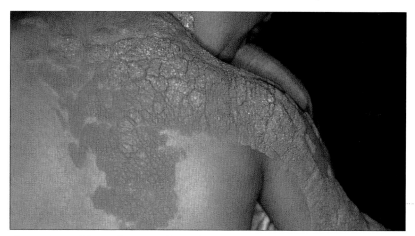

Figure 27. Epidermal nevus. The epidermal nevus represents a localized hyperplasia of epidermal elements. It ranges greatly in size and when large, may follow Blaschko's lines (see **Figure 28**), as shown here. The widely distributed type may be associated with systemic abnormalities of the musculoskeletal, ocular and neurologic systems. (Courtesy of Theodore Sebastian, MD.)

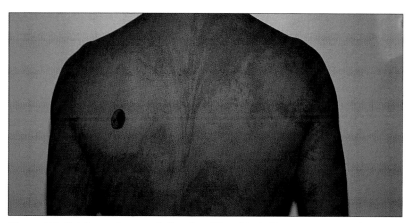

Figure 28. Epidermal nevus following Blaschko's lines. (A tattoo is also seen over the left scapula.) Alfred Blaschko, a private practitioner of dermatology in Berlin, transposed the linear pattern of the skin lesions of more than 140 patients on to dolls and statues. His composite diagram has since been referred to as Blaschko's lines. They are thought to result from the dorsoventral outgrowths of two different cell populations during early embryogenesis. Many congenital skin diseases are distributed according to its pattern.

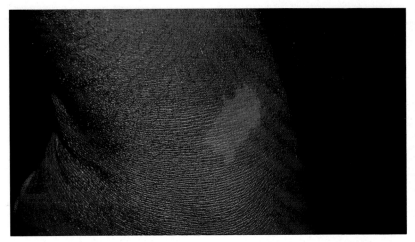

Figure 29. Nevus depigmentosus. A congenital, stable, hypopigmented lesion located randomly, segmentally, linearly or in a whorled fashion is characteristic. Melanocytes are present histologically but do not produce the usual amount of melanin. Wood's light accentuates the lesion. Because some pigment is present perhaps a more accurate name is nevus hypopigmentosus.

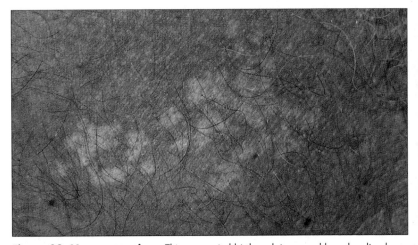

Figure 30. Nevus anemicus. This congenital birthmark is caused by a localized, permanent vasoconstriction of blood vessels. The relative lack of blood gives it a whitish color. There is no alteration of pigment. Its border may be obliterated for several seconds by rubbing a finger across it.

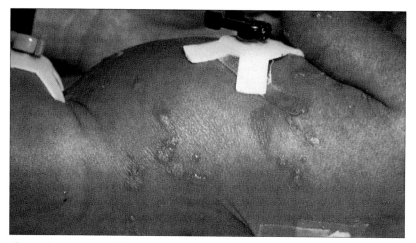

Figure 31. Neonatal herpes. A blistering eruption in a newborn which represents herpes simplex infection is a medical emergency. Transmission may have occurred transplacentally or via the birth canal. Systemic involvement can include encephalitis, pneumonia and hepatitis. (Courtesy of Michael O Murphy, MD.)

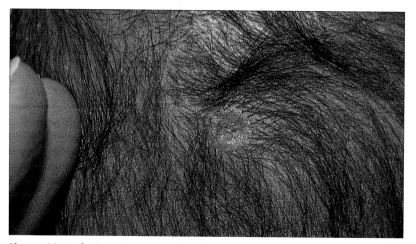

Figure 32. Aplasia cutis congenitia. A congenital, circumscribed area of alopecia and scarring on the scalp is characteristic of aplasia cutis congenita. The presence of dense hair at the periphery (hair collar sign) should raise the possibility of a more significant defect (e.g. rudimentary meningocele).

Infantile Dermatoses

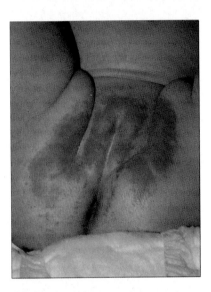

Figure 33. Diaper dermatitis. The diaper area is red and edematous but the flexures are usually spared (in contrast to seborrheic dermatitis, **Figure 35**) in diaper dermatitis. This condition represents an irritant dermatitis from the stool and urine and is worsened by maceration and friction. A bout of diarrhea may bring on or exacerbate the condition.

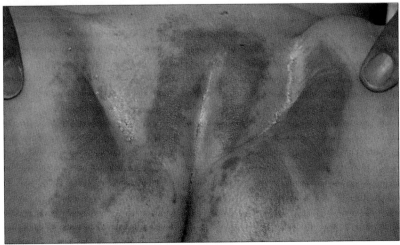

Figure 34. Diaper dermatitis. Note the characteristic sparing of the flexures.

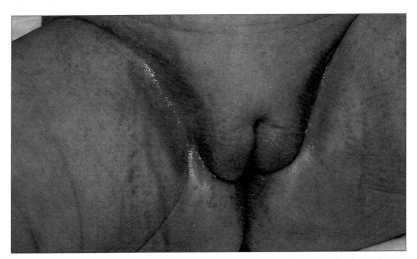

Figure 35. Seborrheic dermatitis, groin. In seborrheic dermatitis of infants, the groin is red and scaly, with prominent involvement of the flexures (in contrast to diaper dermatitis, **Figures 33 and 34**). The scalp is frequently red and scaly. The onset is from 2 weeks to 6 months.

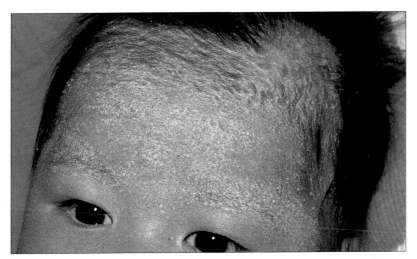

Figure 36. Seborrheic dermatitis, cradle cap. Note the presence of abundant scale in the scalp.

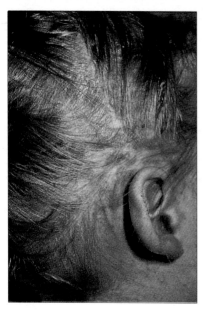

Figure 37. Langerhans' cell histiocytosis, scalp. Langerhans' cell histiocytosis (formerly called histiocytosis X) in an infant may present as a red, scaly, seborrheic dermatitis-like rash of the scalp. Classically, Langerhans' cell histiocytosis has been separated into Letterer–Siwe disease (infants, aggressive, internal involvement), Hand–Schüller–Christian disease (children, bony defects especially of the skull, diabetes insipidus and exophthalmos) and eosinophilic granuloma (children and adults, granulomas of the skin and bones, benign, chronic). Electron microscopy shows a significant number of the cells to contain Birbeck granules, which resemble racquets. (Courtesy of Michael O Murphy, MD.)

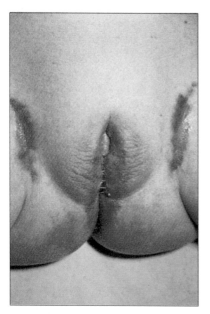

Figure 38. Langerhans' cell histiocytosis, groin. A red, scaly intertrigo-like rash of the groin is characteristic. (Courtesy of Michael O Murphy, MD.)

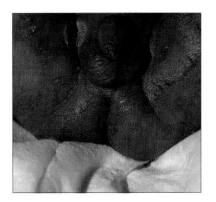

Figure 39. Zinc deficiency, groin. A pustular, bullous and erosive eruption may develop periorally, perianally, acrally and in the genital region in an infant with deficient zinc intake. Infants receiving artificial feeding, or breast-fed infants whose mother's milk is deficient in zinc may be affected. Other diseases that may be associated with a similar rash include acrodermatitis enteropathica, cystic fibrosis, treated maple syrup urine disease, inborn errors of biotin metabolism and neonatal citrullinemia. (Courtesy of James Steger, MD.)

Figure 40. Perianal cellulitis. This disease is characterized by well-demarcated perianal erythema, which may be accompanied by itching, bleeding and painful defecation. The cause is local infection by group A beta hemolytic streptococci. Children aged 7 months to 8 years are most commonly affected.

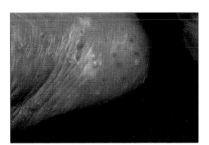

Figure 41. Infantile acropustulosis. Recurrent crops of pruritic pustules on the palms and soles of an infant or young child are characteristic. Both a bacterial infection and scabies infestation should be excluded.

Atopic Dermatitis

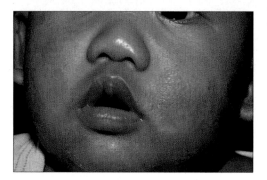

Figure 42. Atopic dermatitis, infantile, cheeks. The patient with atopic dermatitis often has a personal or family history of asthma and/or hay fever. The infant often presents with bilaterally symmetric, red, scaly, chapped and dry, glazed cheeks. An irritant dermatitis from saliva may be contributory.

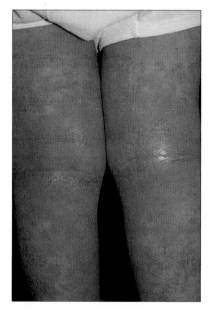

Figure 43. Atopic dermatitis, diffuse, legs. The red, scaly rash of atopic dermatitis may spread to cover much or all of the body. Often there is accentuation of the flexures, as illustrated here. The child scratches incessantly and sleep may be significantly disrupted, both for the child and for the parents.

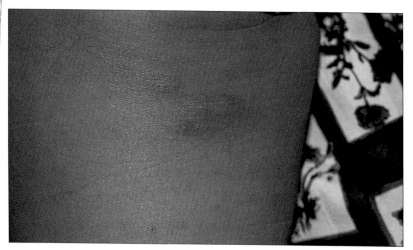

Figure 44. Atopic dermatitis, flexural, posterior, thigh. Areas of the skin commonly affected include the cheeks, neck, antecubital fossa, wrists, popliteal fossa and the upper posterior thigh, as shown here.

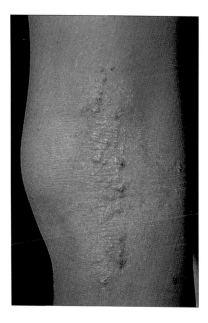

Figure 45. Atopic dermatitis, flexural with lichenification. Much of the skin changes are secondary to scratching. Linear lichenification, as shown here, and excoriations are typical.

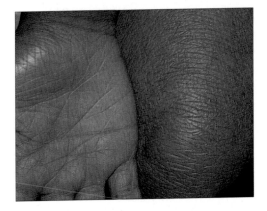

Figure 46. Hyperlinear palms and lichenification, thigh. Atopic patients often develop accentuation of the palmar creases.

Figure 47. Follicular eczema in a Black patient. Dark-skinned patients with atopic dermatitis often show follicular accentuation. At times, only the follicles are involved, as shown here.

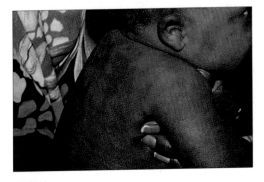

Figure 48. Post-inflammatory hypopigmentation in a Black patient. Temporary hypopigmentation may develop in sites of previous eczema, as shown here. Complete and permanent depigmentation may also develop at sites of chronic disease.

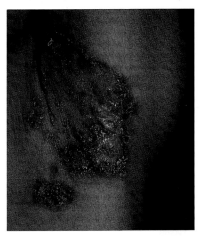

Figure 49. Atopic dermatitis, secondary infection, bacterial. Atopic skin often harbors significant numbers of *Staphylococcus*. Overt infection is common and is manifested by areas of erosion, crusting or oozing, as shown here.

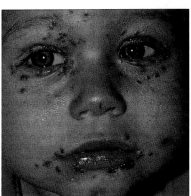

Figure 50. Kaposi's varicelliform eruption, face. The patient with atopic dermatitis is predisposed to infection not only by *Staphylococcus aureus* but also by herpes simplex as shown here. Rapidly progressive, widespread crusted papules, vesicles and erosions are characteristic of this viral infection which most commonly affects the face. (See also **Figure 337**.)

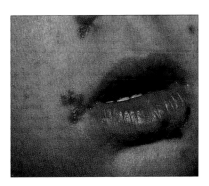

Figure 51. Kaposi's varicelliform eruption, close-up. Crusted lesions in the atopic patient may represent bacterial or viral infection. At times only culture will distinguish the two.

Genodermatoses: Inherited Syndromes

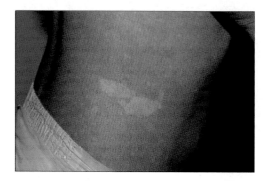

Figure 52. Tuberous sclerosis, ash leaf macule. Tuberous sclerosis is an autosomal dominant disorder that is characterized by skin lesions, mental retardation and seizures. The earliest sign, the ash leaf macule, is usually present in the first year of life. It may appear as a polygonal macule, in the shape of an ash leaf or like confetti. A Wood's light aids in detecting these lesions.

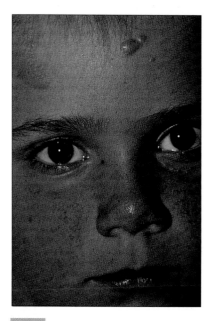

Figure 53. Tuberous sclerosis, adenoma sebaceum and forehead plaque. Sometime during childhood or adolescence, multiple red–yellow papules begin to develop on the face and are called adenoma sebaceum. Firm nodules and plaques on the forehead are also characteristic. Systemic manifestations include cardiac rhabdomyomas, cortical or cerebral tubers, CNS tumors, pulmonary lymphangiomyomatosis, renal angiomyolipomas, renal cysts and retinal astrocytomas.

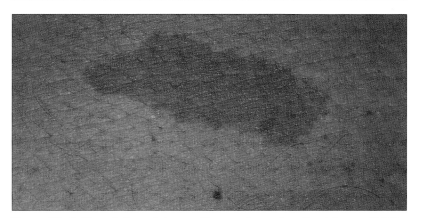

Figure 54. Café-au-lait spot. In neurofibromatosis type 1, café-au-lait spots (CALS) occur with cutaneous neurofibromas. Two of the following seven criteria are important for diagnosis: i) six or more CALS, ii) two or more neurofibromas, iii) Lisch nodules (pigmented iris hamartomas), iv) axillary or groin freckling, v) optic glioma, vi) characteristic bony deformity, and vii) a first-degree relative with two criteria. Systemic abnormalities that may occur in neurofibromatosis include CNS tumors, pheochromocytoma and seizures. Precocious puberty occurs in approximately 3–4% of patients and only in those with tumors of the optic chiasm. Inheritance is autosomal dominant but sporadic cases are common.

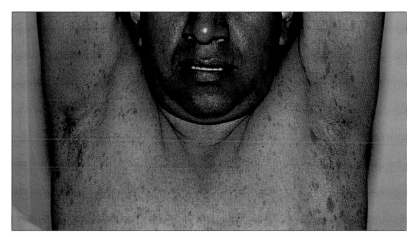

Figure 55. Neurofibromatosis, axillary freckling. Crowe's sign or axillary freckling is characteristic of neurofibromatosis.

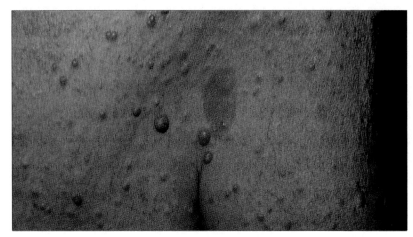

Figure 56. Neurofibromatosis, neurofibromas. Multiple to innumerable neurofibromas develop in neurofibromatosis. A CALS is also seen. Neurofibromas are soft and may be 'button-holed' into the skin.

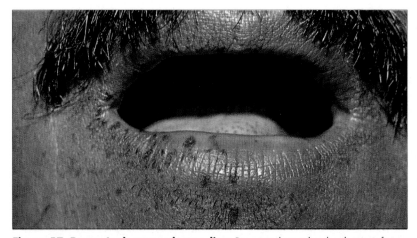

Figure 57. Peutz–Jeghers syndrome, lips. Pigmented macules develop in infancy or early childhood on the lips and buccal mucosa. Gastrointestinal hamartomatous polyps are also associated and develop from the gastroesophageal junction down to the anus, with the small bowel the most commonly affected. Their malignant potential is low. Pigmented macules of the palm, fingers and soles also occur. Inheritance is autosomal dominant.

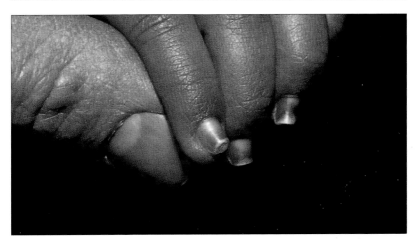

Figure 58. Pachyonychia congenita, nails. All fingers and toenails are greatly thickened, hard and curved transversely in pachyonychia congenita. Inheritance is usually autosomal dominant. The nails illustrated here belong to an affected baby. The doctor's normal thumbnail is shown for comparison.

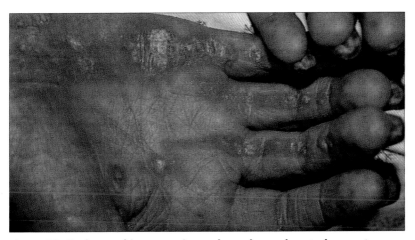

Figure 59. Pachyonychia congenita, palmarplantar keratoderma. A palmarplantar keratoderma is also characteristic of pachyonychia congenita, and is illustrated here. Leukoderma of the oral mucosa and hyperkeratotic papules of the knees and elbows occur. Large friction blisters may form on the palms and soles.

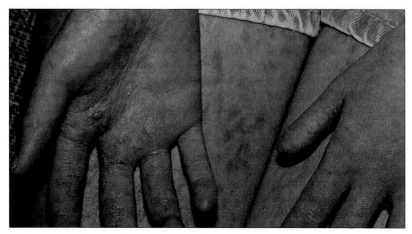

Figure 60. Goltz syndrome. Congenital linear streaks of telangiectasias and atrophy, soft, reddish-yellow nodules (fat herniations) are characteristic of Goltz syndrome (also known as focal dermal hypoplasia). Skeletal abnormalities such as syndactyly, polydactyly and absence of digits occur. Most patients are female.

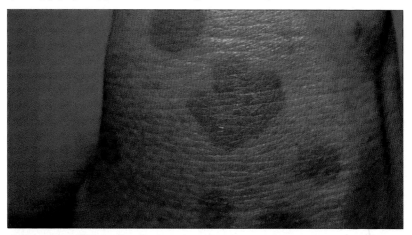

Figure 61. Epidermodysplasia verruciformis, verruca. Epidermodysplasia verruciformis represents an autosomal recessive inherited disease characterized by increased susceptibility to infection by human papilloma virus (HPV), which may be found in the verruca plana lesions (pictured here), tinea versicolor lesions and associated cutaneous malignancies (e.g. Bowen's disease or squamous cell carcinoma). HPV 5 and 8 are the most common types found in these patients. (Courtesy of Steven Goldberg, MD.)

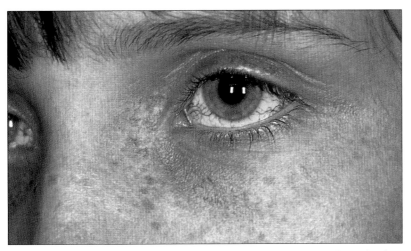

Figure 62. Ataxia telangiectasia. Ocular telangiectasias, as shown here, develop at 3–5 years of age. Ataxia appears when the child tries to walk. Recurrent sinopulmonary infections affect most and bronchiectasis may develop. Telangiectasias develop later on the face (some visible in this patient), ears and elsewhere. There is an increased risk of leukemia or lymphoma. Inheritance is autosomal recessive with variable penetration. (Courtesy of A Götz, MD.)

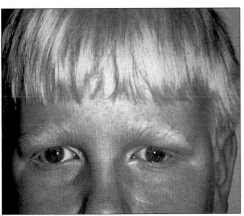

Figure 63. Albinism. The skin is snow white, fair or light tan, the irises may be translucent and the hair white, yellow, light brown or red in oculocutaneous albinism, which comprises a group of disorders with absent or deficient biosynthesis of melanin. These disorders are broadly divided into tyrosine-negative and tyrosine-positive. (Courtesy of James E Rasmussen, MD.)

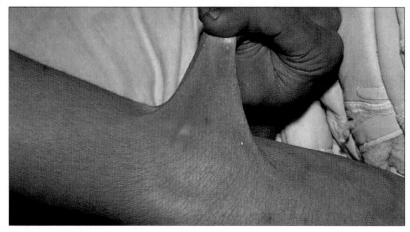

Figure 64. Ehlers–Danlos syndrome, hyperextensible skin. Ehlers–Danlos syndrome is a group of disorders whose main abnormalities include hyperextensible and fragile skin and hyperlaxity of the joints. A specific defect in collagen production has been identified in many of the subtypes. Soft, fleshy papulonodules called molluscoid pseudotumors occur in areas subject to trauma. (Courtesy of Michael O Murphy, MD.)

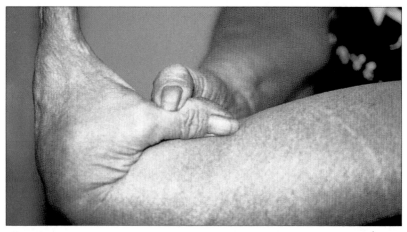

Figure 65. Ehlers–Danlos syndrome, hyperlaxity of the joints. (Courtesy of Theodore Sebastian, MD.)

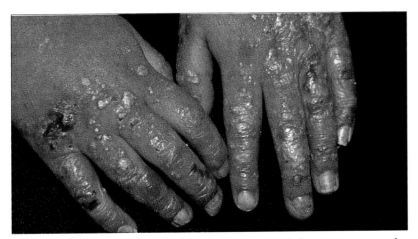

Figure 66. Epidermolysis bullosa, hands. Epidermolysis bullosa (EB) is a group of inherited disorders in which the slightest amount of mechanical trauma can induce blisters and erosions. Three main categories are identified based on the level of separation of the blister: EB simplex (epidermis), junctional EB (basement membrane zone) and dystrophic EB (dermis). The erosions of EB tend to heal slowly with atrophic scarring and milia formation. Multiple milia (small white papules) are seen in the healed areas of this child with EB.

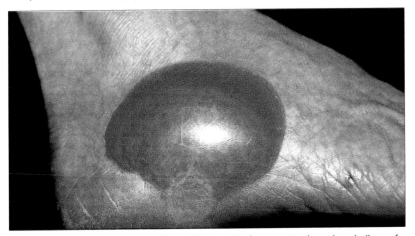

Figure 67. Epidermolysis bullosa, Weber–Cockayne. Epidermolysis bullosa of the Weber–Cockayne subtype has a very mild presentation with blisters confined primarily to the hands and feet. There is no decrease in longevity. Blistering tends to be worse in the summer with increased sweating and friction. The patient pictured is 60 years of age.

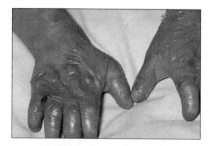

Figure 68. Epidermolysis bullosa, recessive, dystrophic. This is one of the most severe forms of EB. Repeated scarring of the digits leads to flexural contractures, digital fusion and epidermal encasement—the so-called mitten deformity. The nails are lost early in life. In this patient, the skin is scarred, the digits short and the nails absent. (Courtesy of Arlene Tsuchia, MD.)

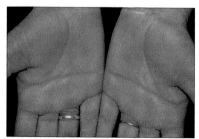

Figure 69. Palmarplantar keratoderma, Unna Thost. A variety of disorders have as part of their presentation uniform keratoderma covering the palms and soles. This patient has the Unna Thost variant, which is inherited as an autosomal dominant condition with no other clinical findings. Note the diffusely hyperkeratotic palms and the margin of erythema.

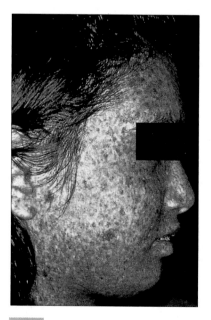

Figure 70. Xeroderma pigmentosum. Extreme sensitivity to ultraviolet rays results from an autosomal recessive inherited defect in the enzymes involved in DNA repair. Erythema and edema after minimal sun exposure develop initially with onset in most patients from 1 to 4 years of age. Later, multiple dark stellate 'freckles' and lentigos (as shown here), telangiectasias and hypopigmented macules develop. Actinic keratoses, basal cell carcinoma, squamous cell carcinoma and melanoma may develop and are a frequent cause of early death. (Courtesy of James Rasmussen, MD.)

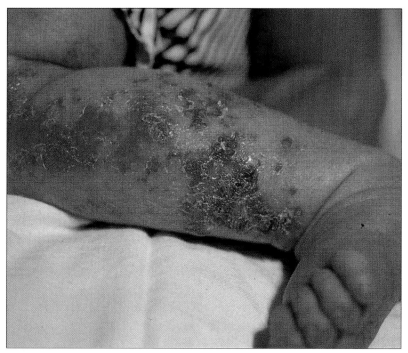

Figure 71. Incontinentia pigmenti, verrucous lesions and erosions. Female infants are affected first by erythematous, vesicular, linear lesions. Soon thereafter, hyperkeratotic linear plaques (shown here) develop that finally resolve leaving linear and whorled hyperpigmentation (see **Figure 72**). The initial vesiculobullous phase is usually present at birth or develops in the first 2 weeks of life, the verrucous second stage from the second to the sixth weeks and the third pigmentary stage is most apparent from 12 to 26 weeks. The pigmentary stage tends to fade and usually does not persist into adulthood. (Courtesy of James Steger, MD.)

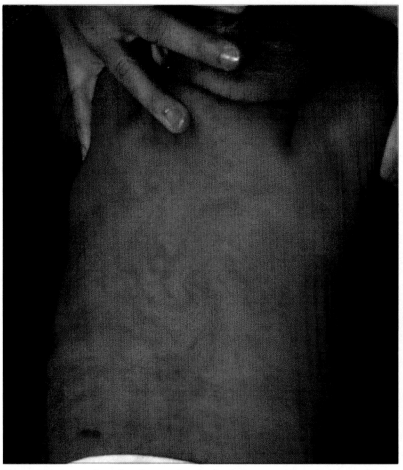

Figure 72. Incontinentia pigmenti, whorled pigmentation. (Courtesy of James Steger, MD.)

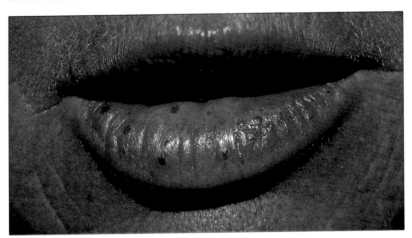

Figure 73. Hereditary hemorrhagic telangiectasias. Also known as Rendu–Osler-Weber syndrome, this autosomal dominant inherited syndrome presents initially with epistaxis in childhood. Later, telangiectatic mats develop on the lips (shown here), tongue, fingertips and elsewhere. Vascular abnormalities of other organs and abscess of the CNS may occur.

Figure 74. Pseudoxanthoma elasticum. Small yellow reticulate papules on the sides of the neck and flexures giving a 'plucked chicken' appearance is characteristic. Onset is in the teenage years. Ophthalmologic and cardiac changes occur. Both mild and severe forms are seen. Inheritance is usually autosomal recessive.

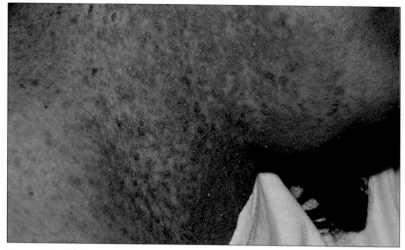

Figure 75. Darier's disease. Also known as keratosis follicularis, Darier's disease presents with scaly, waxy, greasy papules in the seborrheic area, shown here on the neck. It often worsens in the summer and may be aggravated by heat or sunlight. Onset is usually in adolescence with an autosomal dominant inheritance pattern.

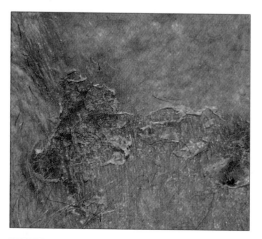

Figure 76. Hailey–Hailey disease. 'Wet tissue paper' erosions or erythematous plaques are found symmetrically in the axilla and groin where the skin surfaces oppose each other in Hailey–Hailey disease, also known as benign familial pemphigus. Inheritance is autosomal dominant with a positive family history approximately 70% of the time.

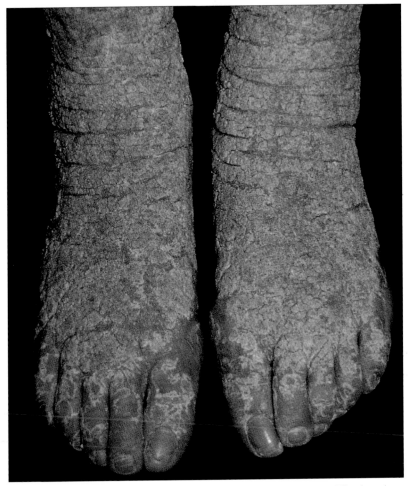

Figure 77. Epidermolytic hyperkeratosis. The affected infant has diffusely red, scaly skin with blister formation (that gave rise to the former name of bullous icthyosiform erythroderma). Later, the skin becomes hyperkeratotic and verrucous diffusely as shown here in this 24-year old woman. Significant palmoplantar keratoderma may occur. This disease is inherited in an autosomal dominant manner.

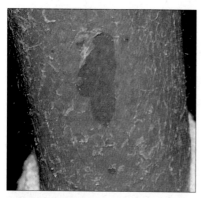

Figure 78. Epidermolytic hyperkeratosis, erosion amongst hyperkeratosis. A very helpful diagnostic sign is areas of denudation and, later, normal skin adjacent to verrucous areas.

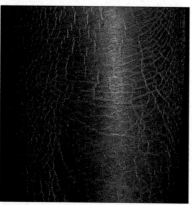

Figure 79. Ichthyosis vulgaris. Normal skin is constantly turning over, with the old cells coming to the surface and being shed. In the ichthyoses, this process is abnormal and thickened, scaly or hyperkeratotic skin results. The most common and the most mild of the ichthyoses is ichthyosis vulgaris. This autosomal dominant inherited disease is most prominent on the legs and worsens in the winter. An important feature histologically is an absence of the granular layer.

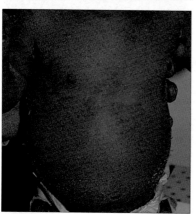

Figure 80. Congenital ichthyosiform erythroderma. The skin is diffusely erythematous with fine scaling in this autosomal recessive inherited ichthyosis.

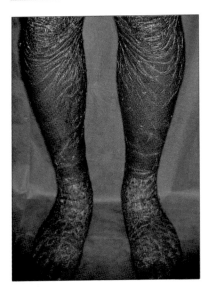

Figure 81. Lamellar ichthyosis.
Lamellar ichthyosis often presents as a collodion baby at birth. Later, the skin becomes ichthyotic with large plate-like scales and variable erythroderma. Ectropion and palmarplantar keratoderma are frequently present. Inheritance is autosomal recessive. (Courtesy of Department of Dermatology, UCSD.)

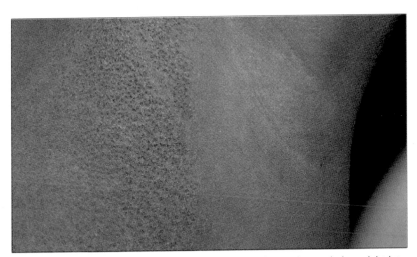

Figure 82. Recessive X-linked ichthyosis. The scales are large, dark, and thick in this condition. The flexures are typically spared, as illustrated here. Corneal opacities may be found. Cryptorchidism and testicular cancer unassociated with cryptorchidism may occur. Only males are affected, although carrier females may exhibit mild features as well as failure to go into labor spontaneously.

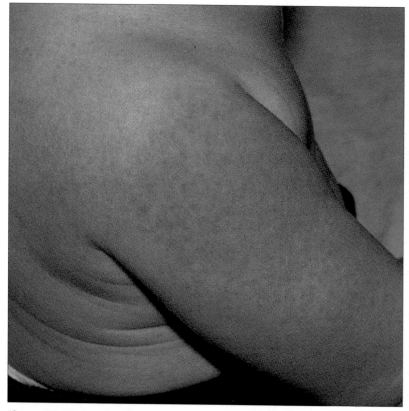

Figure 83. Keratosis pilaris, arms. In this very common disease, tiny, 1 mm, follicular hyperkeratotic papules with or without erythema are found on the upper, outer arms. The anterior thighs, buttocks and cheeks may also be affected and a diffuse truncal eruption may rarely occur. Why the hair follicles become 'clogged' and at times inflamed is unknown.

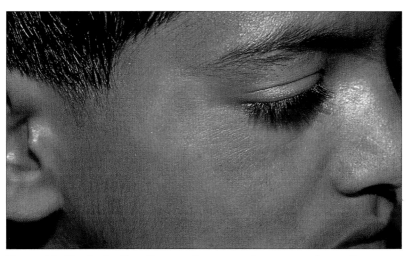

Figure 84. Pityriasis alba. Pityriasis alba seems to be a variant of post-inflammatory hypopigmentation. The initial event is a patch of eczema, which may or may not be noticed. The child then presents with multiple, hypopigmented, ill-defined areas on the face and/or arms. Often there is a history of atopic dermatitis.

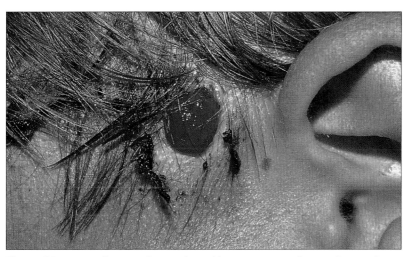

Figure 85. Pyogenic granuloma. The sudden appearance of a vascular papule that bleeds easily on the finger, palm, sole, head or neck is characteristic of a pyogenic granuloma. Patients may apply layer upon layer of bandages to control the bleeding giving rise to the 'bandage sign'.

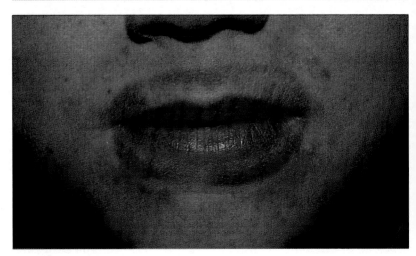

Figure 86. Liplicking. Red, scaly, crusted, eczematous changes of the skin encircling the mouth in a child are characteristic. Only skin accessible to the tongue is affected. This represents an irritant contact dermatitis from the constant wetting and irritation by the saliva.

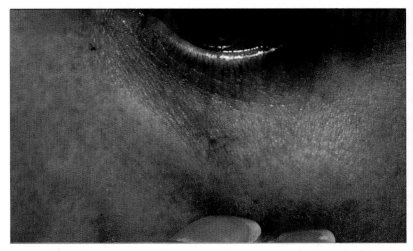

Figure 87. Spider angioma. The area just below the eye on the upper cheek is a very characteristic site for spider telangiectasias in children. An arcade of vessels radiating out from a central arteriole is the characteristic appearance. Compressing the central point blanches the arcade. It is very common in children, in pregnancy and with liver disease.

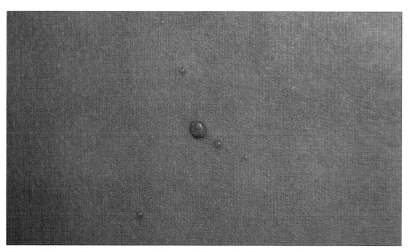

Figure 88. Molluscum contagiosum. This viral infection is akin to warts but tends to affect only specific groups of patients. Children 2–6 years of age may present with 2–50 lesions scattered all over the body. They are pink-to-flesh-colored, smooth papules with a central dell (brought out nicely during cryotherapy). Affected children often have a history of spending much time in the swimming pool. Molluscum may also affect patients with atopic dermatitis, adults as an STD (**Figure 318**) or patients infected with HIV (**Figures 261 and 262**).

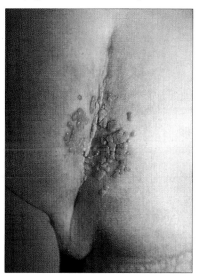

Figure 89. Condyloma, perianal. The possibility of sexual abuse must be considered and is more likely if the child is 3 years old or older. Younger children are more likely to have received the virus from the mother during pregnancy and/or delivery. Alternative modes of inoculation include transfer from the patient's own or a parent's hand warts. (Courtesy of Michael O Murphy, MD.)

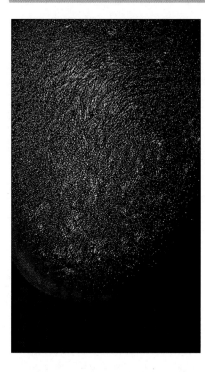

Figures 90–93. Tinea capitis. Tinea capitis may present clinically in various ways including diffuse scale resembling seborrheic dermatitis (**Figure 90**, left), a circumscribed area of alopecia with thick crust (**Figure 91**, below), a boggy mass of tissue (kerion, **Figure 92**, right), multiple hairs broken off at the level of the scalp (black dot ringworm, **Figure 93**, below right), yellow cup-shaped crusts (scutula) each pierced by a hair (also known as favus) and scattered, patchy areas of alopecia with slight scale. Note the regional lymphadenopathy in **Figure 92** that results from the tremendous inflammatory response. Wood's light fluorescence is positive in some patients. Prepubescent children are usually affected. In the USA, crowded living conditions and urban areas are risk factors. A high percentage of siblings, parents and grandparents of the index patients are asymptomatic carriers. Most cases in the USA are caused by *Trichophyton tonsurans*.

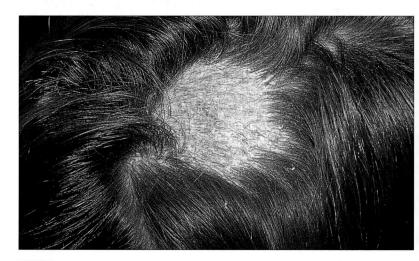

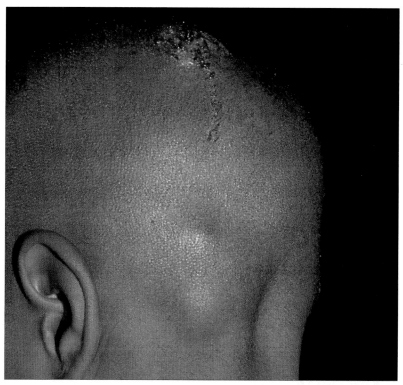

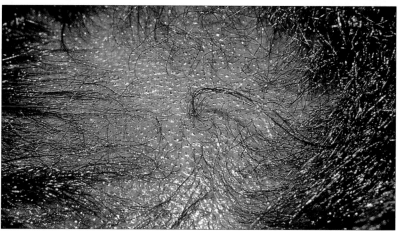

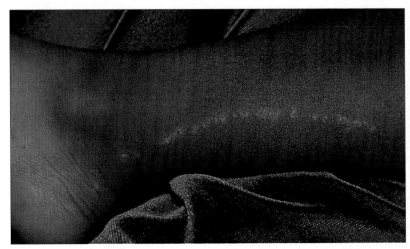

Figure 94. Lichen striatus. In this benign inflammatory condition of unknown cause, linear papules or red, scaly lesions appear suddenly in a child and follow Blaschko's lines. In a series of 18 patients with lichen striatus, the mean age of onset was 3 years, mean duration 9.5 months and hypochromic sequelae occurred in 50%. If the proximal nail fold is involved, nail dystrophy may occur.

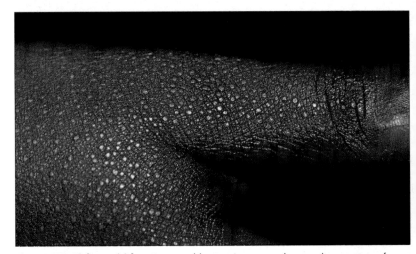

Figure 95. Lichen nitidus. Innumerable, tiny 1 mm papules are characteristic of lichen nitidus. Many sites may be affected.

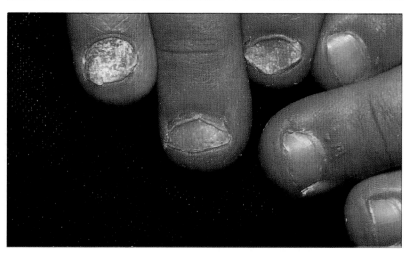

Figure 96. Trachyonychia. Only a few to all finger and toe nails may become rough or ridged in trachyonychia. When all the nails are affected, the term 20-nail dystrophy may be used. Trachyonychia is usually idiopathic but may occur in association with alopecia areata, psoriasis, or lichen planus.

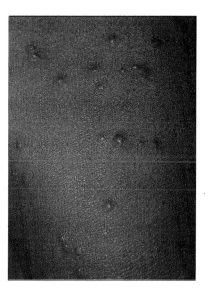

Figure 97. Flea bites. A child will present with multiple, scattered, pruritic papules. The larger the child, the more the lesions are localized to the lower leg. Vesicles and bulla may occur. (See also **Figure 377**.)

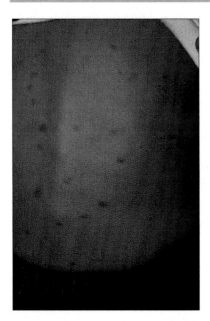

Figure 98. Uriticaria pigmentosa.
Various patterns of cutaneous mastocytosis occur. In urticaria pigmentosa, multiple, brown macules or papules occur, scattered on the body. Patients may have a few to several thousand. The trunk is the most common site, followed by the extremities. Gastrointestinal or systemic histamine effects include diarrhea, stomach pain, flushing or lightheadedness.

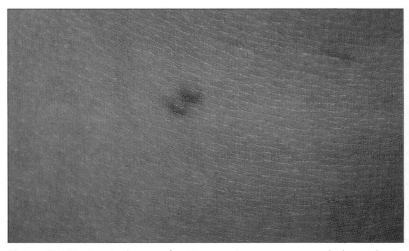

Figure 99. Mastocytosis, papule. Mastocytosis may present as multiple papules, in this case in a child.

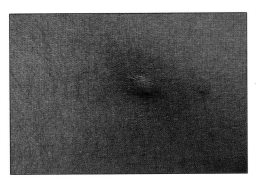

Figure 100. Mastocytosis, Darier's sign. Stroking a papule causes urtication, also known as Darier's sign. (See also **Figures 22 and 656**.)

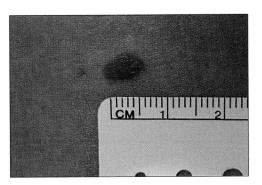

Figure 101. Spitz nevus. A smooth, firm, red-to-brown papulonodule on the cheek of a child is most characteristic but any age or body site may be affected. Some are highly vascular and mimic a hemangioma or a pyogenic granuloma. Histologic differentiation from melanoma may be difficult in some patients.

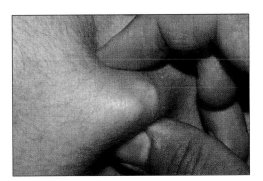

Figure 102. Pilomatricoma. A hard, irregular, dermal or subcutaneous tumor in a child, often on the head or neck, is characteristic. It may be multiple and familial or rarely associated with myotonic dystrophy. When the skin is stretched over the skin, as shown here, multiple nodularities may be seen—the so-called tent sign.

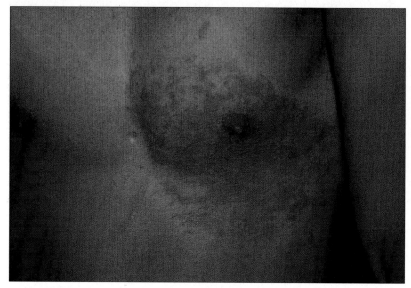

Figure 103. Becker's nevus. An acquired, unilateral, pigmented patch with irregular borders on the trunk of an adolescent is characteristic of a Becker's nevus. Hypertrichosis may develop later, and familial cases have occurred. Breast hypoplasia has occurred in lesions overlying a woman's breast.

See also Verruca, **Figures 348–356**.

Childhood Rashes

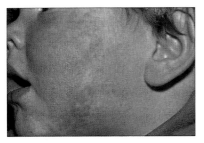
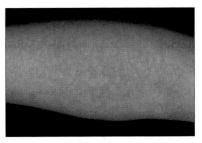

Figures 104 and 105. Erythema infectiosum. In this infection by Parvovirus B19, a child will develop prominent erythema of the cheeks ('slapped cheeks', **Figure 104**, left) followed by a lace-like erythema on the extremities (**Figure 105**, right) and buttocks. A sore throat, cough, headache, nausea and fever may accompany the rash. It is also known as fifth's disease.

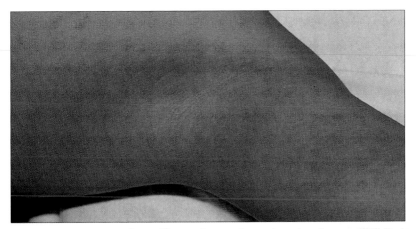

Figure 106. Asymmetric periflexural exanthem. A scarlatiniform or eczematous eruption unilaterally on the lateral trunk and/or axilla of a child is characteristic. The age of onset is typically 1–3 years of age, with girls affected more often than boys. It may also begin in the inguinal folds, and the regional lymph nodes may be moderately enlarged. A mild fever may be present. Later, it may spread e.g. to the other side of the thorax, the elbows, knees and thighs creating a symmetric distribution.

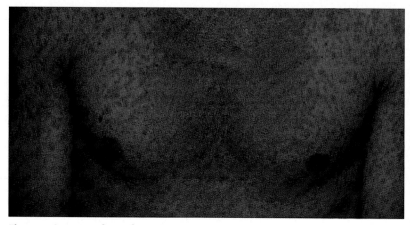

Figure 107. Measles. After an incubation period of 10–12 days and a prodrome of fever, malaise, coryza, conjunctivitis and cough, the patient will develop a maculopapular rash starting on the face and progressing to involve the trunk and extremities by the third day. Punctate whitish spots like salt grains on a red base on the buccal mucosa (Koplick's spots) are classic, developing in the prodromal period and disappearing by the height of the exanthem. Measles is caused by an RNA parmyxovirus.

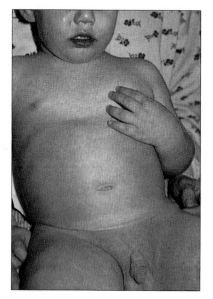

Figure 108. Kawasaki disease. Five of the following six criteria are necessary for diagnosis: i) fever for 5 days or more unresponsive to antibiotics, ii) bilateral 'dry' conjunctival congestion, iii) oral mucosal changes (e.g. red, crusted lips, strawberry tongue), iv) palmar/plantar changes (e.g. erythema and edema with characteristic desquamation later), v) polymorphous exanthem (e.g. maculopapular, scarlatiniform, erythema multiforme-like), and vi) cervical lymphadenopathy (relatively non-tender). The patient is usually a young child. Approximately 20–25% of untreated patients develop significant cardiovascular complications including arrythmias (acute), aneurysms and thrombi (subacute) or scarring and ischemic heart disease (late). (Courtesy of Lon Dubey, MD.)

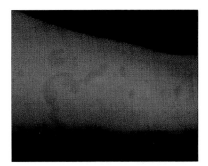

Figure 109. Urticaria. Urticaria in children less than 6 months is commonly caused by allergy to cow's milk. For children 6–24 months, a drug (e.g. ASA, amoxicillin) or a viral illness (e.g. hepatitis) is the most common cause. Other potential allergens in children are foods (e.g. milk, peanuts, seafood, eggs), insect bites (e.g. bees, wasps) and bacterial infection (e.g. *Streptococcus*). (See also **Figures 647 and 648**.)

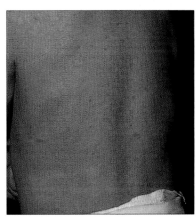

Figure 110. Roseola. The infant 6–18 months of age will develop a high fever but seems relatively well. Then as the fever breaks, multiple pale pink 1–5 mm macules and papules appear and last only hours to a few days. This syndrome also known as exanthem subitum, is caused by human herpes virus 6, human herpes virus 7, and possibly other agents.

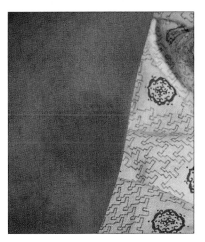

Figure 111. Urticarial vasculitis. Urticarial vasculitis is not a specific disease but instead a clinical finding that is usually associated with a vasculitis that causes significant permeability of the dermal microvasculature. A search for a causative antigen should be undertaken. This child's lesions were fixed and contained a central area of purpura, distinguishing them from urticaria.

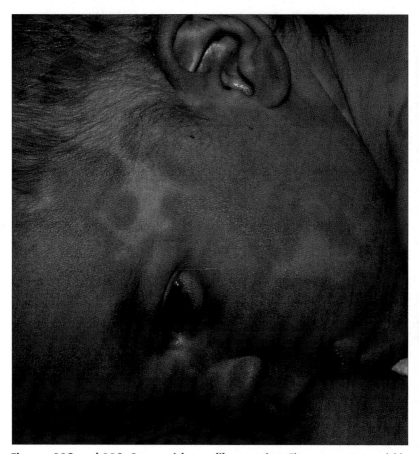

Figures 112 and 113. Serum sickness-like reaction. The acute onset in a child of inflammatory, red papulonodules that spread out into annular, urticarial plaques with dusky centers ('purple urticaria') is characteristic. The onset is usually 7–10 days after the causative drug was begun. There are no true target lesions as with erythema multiforme and the lesions are fixed (other than the fact that they expand) unlike urticaria. The child often has joint pains and fever. Lymphadenopathy and renal involvement usually do not occur in contrast to a true serum sickness. It has occurred most frequently after treatment with cefaclor but may occur with other cephalosporins, penicillins or other drugs.

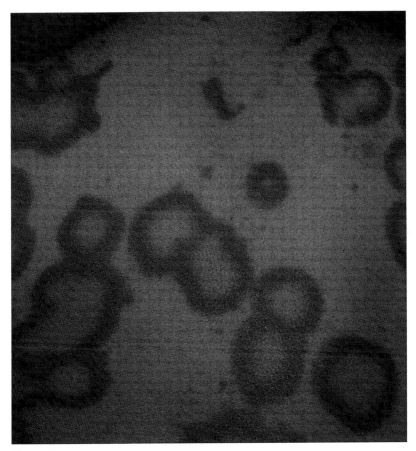

Figure 113.

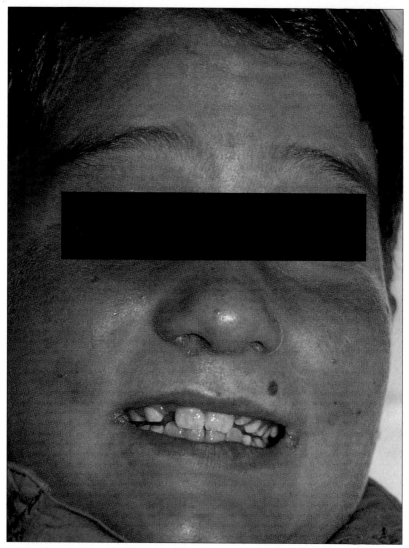

Figure 114. Juvenile dermatomyositis. Juvenile dermatomyositis is characterized by progressive muscle weakness, an erythematous rash of the face and elsewhere and calcification of soft tissue. Unlike adults, the coexistence of cancer is rare. A vasculitis of the gastrointestinal tract and myocardium may occur. (See also **Figures 201 and 202**.)

Figures 115 and 116. Scarlet fever.
A child typically 4–8 years of age will develop a high fever, sore throat, headache and vomiting. The exanthem follows within 1–2 days and appears as many small papules on diffuse erythema (**Figure 115**, left). The skin may feel rough like sandpaper. Linear petechiae in the axilla and groin—Pastia's lines—are classic, as is circumoral palor. Desquamation, worse on the hands and feet, begins 7–10 days later (**Figure 116**, below). The tongue may be initially white and later red (strawberry tongue). The rash of scarlet fever is caused by a toxin-producing group A beta hemolytic *Streptococcus*. The tonsil or pharynx is the usual site of infection but surgical wounds or other foci are possible.

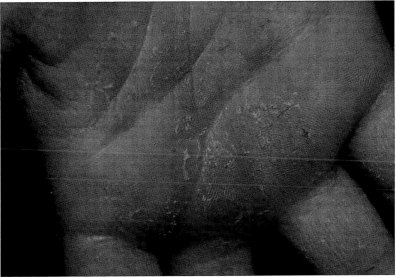

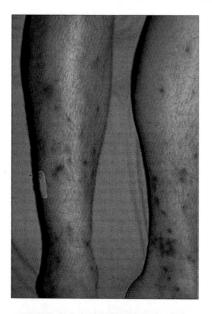

Figure 117. Henoch–Schönlein purpura. A child, 3–10 years of age, who develops palpable purpura on the legs and buttocks, along with abdominal pain, vomiting, diarrhea, melena, hematuria and arthralgias is characteristic. Significant knee and ankle swelling may occur. At times, edematous, urticarial, necrotic or hemangioma-like lesions may occur. Viral or bacterial infections, food or drugs are thought to be triggering events. IgA deposits may be seen on direct immunofluorescence, although this test may not be worth doing, especially in a child. (See also **Figure 679**.) (Courtesy of James Rasmussen, MD.)

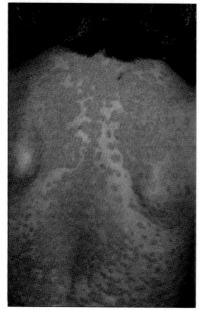

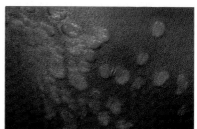

Figures 118 (left) **and 119** (above). **Guttate psoriasis.** This type of psoriasis is the most common type in children and is characterized by the sudden development of disseminated 0.5–2.0 cm, red, scaly papules or small plaques. An upper respiratory tract infection is a very common precipitant. The disease may remit spontaneously or proceed to chronic plaque-type psoriasis. Both children pictured here are 5 years of age. Note the residual post-inflammatory hypopigmentation in **Figure 119**. (See also **Figure 504**.)

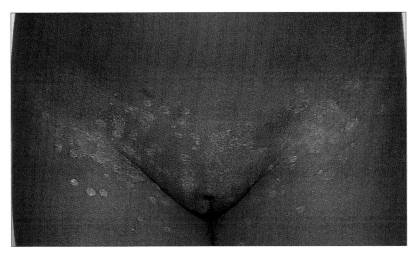

Figure 120. Pityriasis rosea. The papulosquamous papules and plaques of pityriasis rosea commonly affect children and young adults. The groin is a preferred site as illustrated in this 5-year-old girl. (See also **Figures 519–523**.)

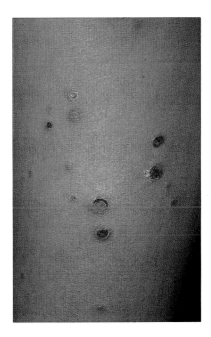

Figure 121. PLEVA. PLEVA is an acronym for pityriasis lichenoides et varioliformis acuta. The characteristic lesion is initially a red papule that develops a hemorrhagic and necrotic center. Lesions of all stages occur and are illustrated on this child's leg. Fever and constitutional symptoms may accompany the outbreak.

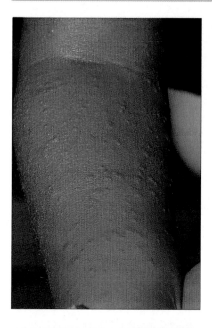

Figure 122. Gianotti–Crosti syndrome. This rash seems to result from an underlying viral infection. It may occur in association with hepatitis B, varicella, coxsackie and Epstein–Barr viruses. The patient acutely develops hundreds of red macules and papules on the face, extremities and buttocks with sparing of the trunk.

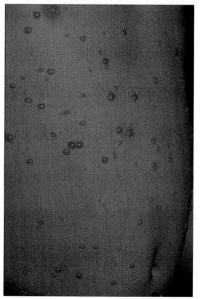

Figure 123. Chickenpox. The varicella zoster virus causes both chickenpox (varicella) and shingles (herpes zoster). The child develops crops of several to hundreds of vesicles, each like a drop of water on an erythematous base on the trunk, face, extremities and oral mucosa. Headache, malaise and fever may accompany the rash. Systemic involvement is more common in adults and may consist of pneumonia, hepatitis, glomerulonephritis, encephalitis and arthritis.

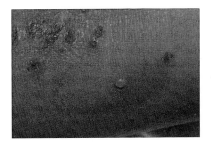

Figure 124. Bullous impetigo.
Cutaneous infection by *Staphylococcus aureus* causes inflammation and a honey-colored crust (see **Figure 49**). If an epidermolytic toxin is produced by the bacteria, vesicles and bullae may form, as shown here.

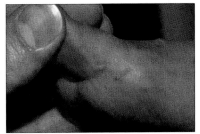

Figure 125. Hand, foot and mouth disease. This viral infection (usually by coxsackie A-16) of young children can produce 3–8 mm. gray–white oval vesicles on the hands, feet and buttocks. Aphthae-like erosions occur in the mouth. A low grade fever, malaise and lymphadenopathy may be seen. Epidemics are common.

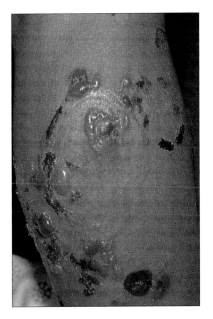

Figure 126. Chronic bullous disease of childhood. Large bullae, often in rosettes or in clusters of 'jewels' in a prepubertal child, are characteristic of this disease. The perioral and genital area are often affected. Direct immuno-fluorescence shows linear IgA along the basement membrane zone. Unlike dermatitis herpetiformis, a gluten-sensitive enteropathy is not associated.

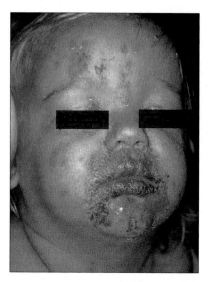

Figure 127. Staphylococcal scalded skin syndrome. A localized infection of *Staphylococcus aureus* causes this disease. The bacteria secrete an exfoliating toxin that causes the skin at sites distant from the infection to become erythematous and tender. Superficial desquamation follows, at times in large sheets. The face may be heavily involved (looking like someone hit the patient in the face with an 'impetigo pie'). Toxic epidermal necrosis should be excluded (see **Figure 219**). (Courtesy of Eliot Mostow, MD.)

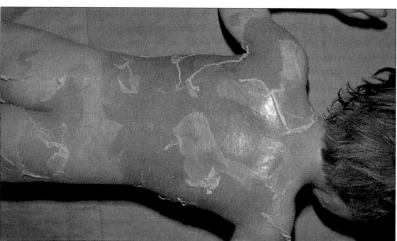

Figure 128. Staphylococcal scalded skin syndrome. Widespread desquamation is seen. (Courtesy of James Rasmussen, MD.)

For related diseases, see also herpes zoster in a child, **Figure 344**.

Section 3

Adult Dermatology

Acne and Related Conditions

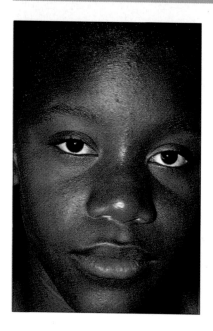

Figure 129. Acne vulgaris, early.
Classic teenage acne begins around age 10–14 years as open and closed comedones (blackheads and whiteheads, respectively) of the central face. Increased sebum production, proliferation of *Propionibacterium acnes* and abnormal keratinization of the follicular epithelium are the principal contributory factors.

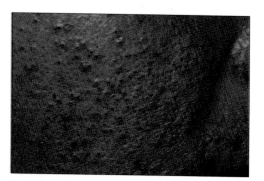

Figure 130. Acne vulgaris, open comedones. The opening of the follicle is clogged by lipid and cellular debris. The black color of open comedones represents melanin (not dirt!).

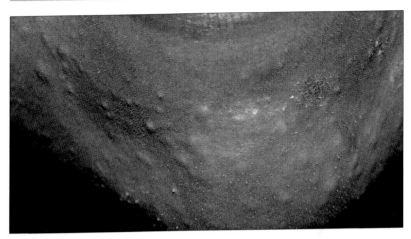

Figure 131. Acne vulgaris, closed comedones. The small white papules on this woman's chin represent closed comedones. They are usually not very apparent unless the skin is stretched, as shown here.

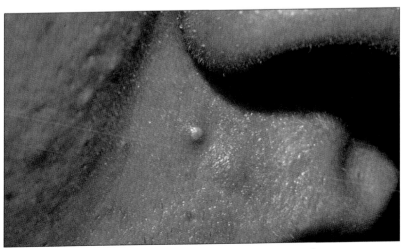

Figure 132. Acne vulgaris, pustular. Mounting pressure and inflammation can rupture the follicle, extruding its inflammatory contents into the dermis. This process converts a non-inflammatory comedone to an inflammatory papule, pustule or nodule.

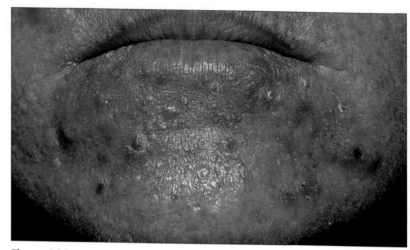

Figure 133. Acne vulgaris, papulopustular, scarring. Deep, inflammatory papules and nodules can cause significant scarring. Young adult women, as the one pictured here, are commonly afflicted along the jaw line and chin.

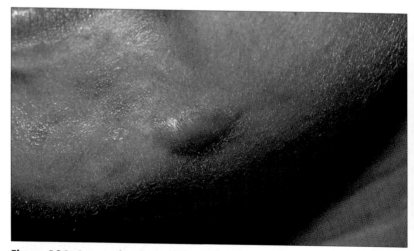

Figure 134. Acne vulgaris, nodulocystic. Ruptured follicular contents and an associated intense inflammatory response can cause extensive tissue destruction. An acne 'cyst' may result. The 'cystic' acne lesion is not a true cyst as it lacks an epithelial wall. The bulging abscess may be fluctuant but incision and drainage causes additional scarring.

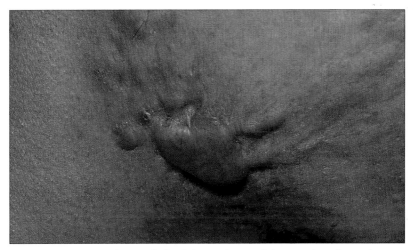

Figure 135. Acne vulgaris, keloidal scarring. Both large and small acne lesions can produce significant scarring. Scars may be atrophic, 'ice pick', hypertrophic or keloidal, as shown here.

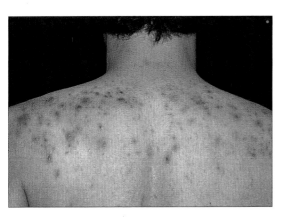

Figure 136. Acne vulgaris, back. The upper back is a common site for acne, especially in young adult men. Erythematous papules and nodules predominate and comedones are inconspicuous. Mechanical factors may play an etiologic role. This variant tends to respond less well to therapy.

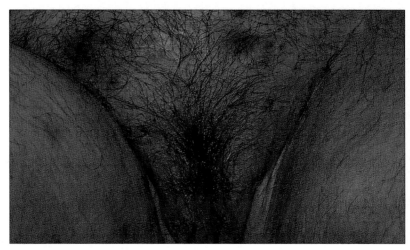

Figure 137. Hidradenitis suppurativa, groin. Hidradenitis suppurativa, acne conglobata and dissecting cellulitis of the scalp represent the follicular occlusion triad. Some add the pilonidal sinus to make a tetrad. These conditions may occur alone or in combination in the same patient. This woman suffered from repeated bouts of inflammatory nodules of the groin and infra-mammary area.

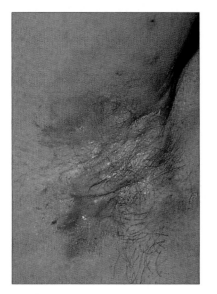

Figure 138. Hidradenitis suppurativa, axilla. Despite its name and the fact that hidradenitis suppurativa affects areas inhabited by apocrine glands, it appears to be caused by poral occlusion of the pilosebaceous unit with inflammation of the apocrine glands occurring secondarily. Patients will present with inflammatory nodules and sterile abscesses of the axilla, the groin, infra-mammary area,and/or the perianal area. Later, with chronic inflammation, sinus tracts, fistulas and hypertrophic scarring develop, as shown here.

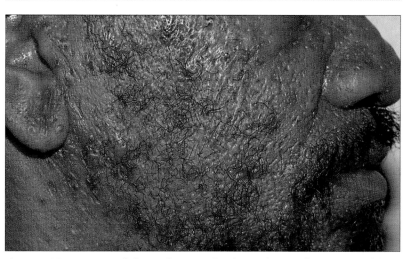

Figure 139. Acne conglobata, face. Fistulated comedones, inflammatory nodules with pus, scarring and sinus tracts of the back, buttocks, face and chest occur in acne conglobata. This disease most commonly affects young males. The dividing line between severe acne and acne conglobata is not always clear.

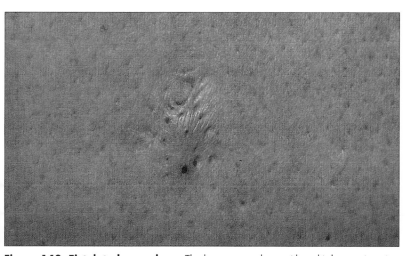

Figure 140. Fistulated comedone. The larger comedone with multiple openings is characteristic of acne conglobata and occurs in greatest numbers on the back. It actually forms by multiple sebaceous follicles merging via an inflammatory process, and represents a scar. The only effective treatment of this lesion is unroofing the cavity.

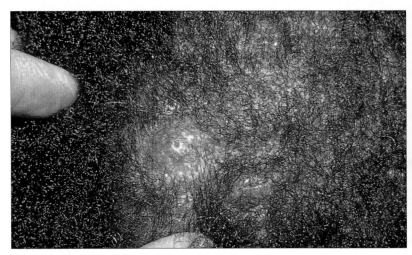

Figure 141. Dissecting cellulitis of the scalp. Inflammatory nodules, sinus tracts, chronic drainage and sclerosing alopecia occur in this disease, also known as perifolliculitis capitis abscedens et suffodiens. Tufts of hair may emanate from a single opening.

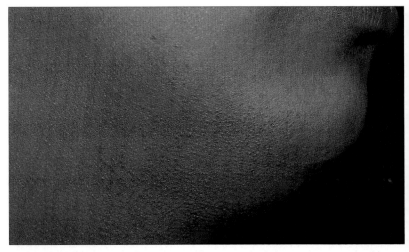

Figure 142. Hirsutism. The presence of excessive body hair in a woman should suggest the possibility of an endocrinologic abnormality playing a role in the patient's acne. Menstrual abnormalities and androgenic alopecia may also be found. This woman shaves in order to control her condition.

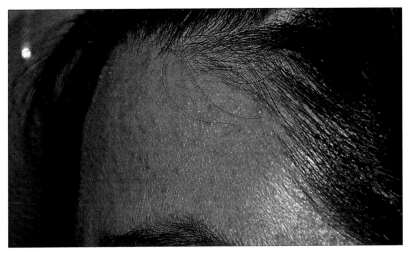

Figure 143. Pomade acne. When the acne is concentrated on the forehead and/or temples, the possibility of greasy, comedogenic hair substances should be entertained. Mousses, gels and conditioners are common offenders.

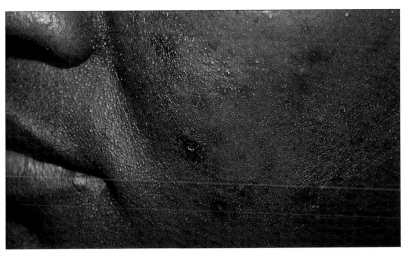

Figure 144. Post-inflammatory hyperpigmentation. Dark-skinned patients frequently develop hyperpigmented macules at the sites of previous acne lesions.

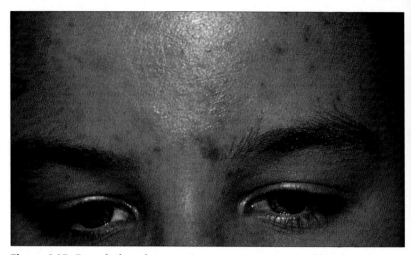

Figure 145. Excoriations in acne. Some acne patients are unable to keep their hands away from their face. Multiple excoriations are the result. The physician can learn quickly to recognize these patients by the large red spots their fingernails leave, as shown here on the glabella. Patients with no underlying acne but who still scratch their face must be excluded.

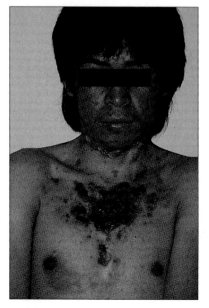

Figure 146. Acne fulminans. White boys, aged 13–16 years of age are most commonly affected. They usually have a history of mild acne but present with the acute onset of inflammatory nodules on the chest and back that may break down leaving crusted ulcerations. Virtually all patients complain of fever, arthralgias and myalgias. Bone pain is common and osseous defects may be present.

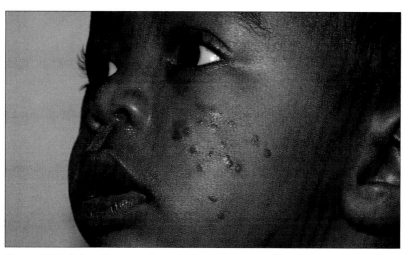

Figure 147. Infantile acne. The typical manifestations of acne may occur rarely in a child, usually male with onset usually from 3 to 6 months. The face is primarily affected with comedones, small papules, pustules and even deep-seated papules and nodules. Congenital adrenal hyperplasia or a virilizing tumor should be excluded.

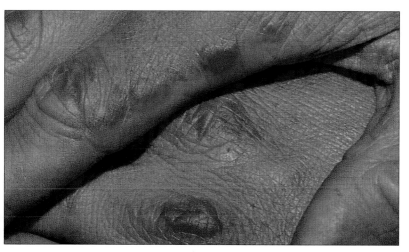

Figure 148. Photodermatitis, doxycycline. Doxycycline is known for its ability to cause significant sun sensitivity. The nose and back of the hands are most commonly affected by confluent erythema and, when severe, blistering as shown here.

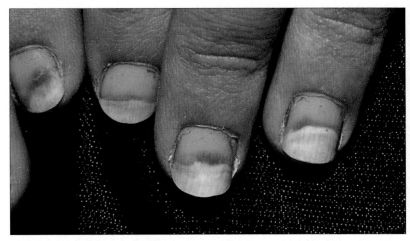

Figure 149. Photo-onycholysis, tetracycline. Patients on tetracycline who receive significant sun exposure may develop a phototoxic reaction of the nailbed, causing the nail plate to separate. Most if not all of the finger nails are usually affected.

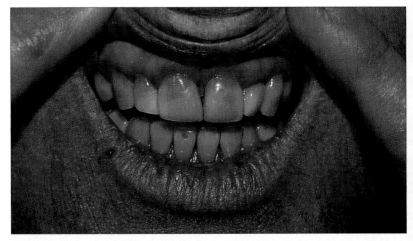

Figure 150. Minocycline pigmentation, teeth. Chronic minocycline therapy can cause various parts of the body to turn blue, including the teeth, nails, scars and skin. Both facial acne scars as well as scars from other trauma may be affected. Patients on higher doses, e.g. 100 mg twice a day, are at greatest risk. This patient had been on minocycline for 15 years.

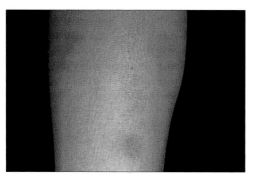

Figure 151. Minocycline pigmentation, legs. These patches are usually thought by the patient to be bruises and in fact they probably started out that way. The color, however, is too blue and persistent. The pigment deposition is composed primarily of minocycline and iron.

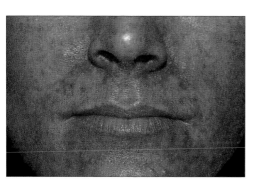

Figure 152. Periorificial dermatitis. Tiny erythematous papules, pustules and a small amount of scale occur about the mouth in periorificial dermatitis, which typically affects young women. Confluent erythema of the nasolabial fold is a classic sign and a narrow zone about the lips is typically spared. The use of a potent topical steroid may trigger or contribute to the eruption. Comedones are absent.

Figure 153. Steroid acne. Steroid acne usually begins several weeks after the administration of systemic corticosteroids. Follicular papules and pustules develop primarily on the trunk. The lesions tend to be monomorphous and comedones are usually absent.

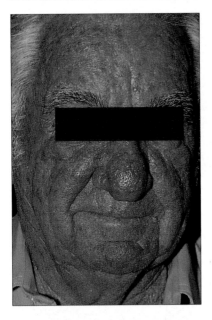

Figures 154 (left) **and 155** (below). **Rosacea.** The nose is red. Erythematous papules and occasional pustules are scattered symmetrically on the face. Comedones are absent. Telangiectasias may accumulate over time and ocular involvement may occur. It is most common in the middle-aged and the fair-skinned. Many patients have a significant flush or blush of the cheeks that may be precipitated by hot liquids.

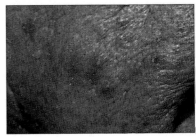

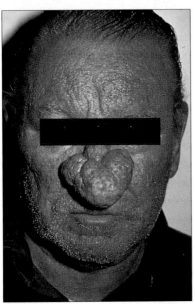

Figure 156. Rhinophyma. In advanced stages of rosacea, significant and disfiguring dermal hypertrophy may occur. The most common of these swellings or 'phymas' is rhinophyma, as pictured here. (Courtesy of Michael O Murphy, MD.)

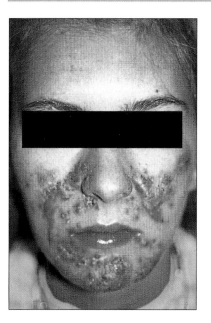

Figure 157. Rosacea fulminans.
The acute onset of large, deep, inflammatory nodules and abscess on the face of a young adult woman is characteristic of rosacea fulminans, formerly called pyoderma faciale. The chin, cheeks and forehead are preferentially affected. Absent are constitutional symptoms (in contrast to acne fulminans), comedones and typical acne lesions on the chest and back. (Courtesy of Theodore Sebastian, MD.)

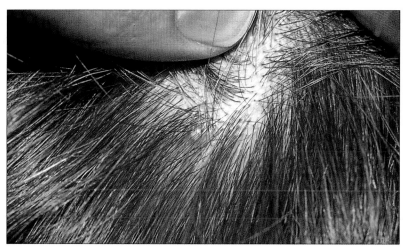

Figure 158. Acne necrotica. Multiple small pustules of the scalp in a middle-aged man are classic for this disease. Pruritus may be significant. The lesions may rupture quickly to leave crusted scabs, which are often picked. Facial lesions along the hairline also occur.

Allergic Contact Dermatitis

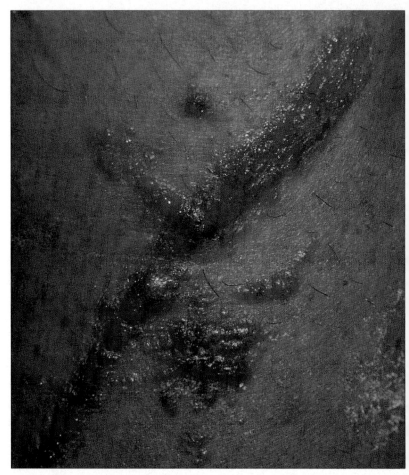

Figure 159. Rhus dermatitis. The classic appearance of allergic contact dermatitis is illustrated in this patient who came into contact with poison oak. The lesions are linear but do not follow Blaschko's lines. The eruption is microvesicular and extremely pruritic.

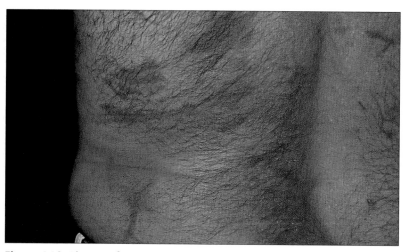

Figure 160. Fig tree dermatitis. This patient was pruning a fig tree without a shirt. The lesions are linear and haphazardly arranged. The area on the lower left suggests a liquid allergen ran down the back.

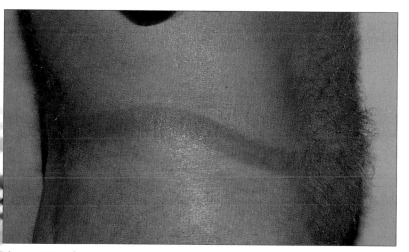

Figure 161. Elastic (waist band) dermatitis. This red, pruritic eruption is unmistakably related to elastic in the patient's underwear. The eruption did not develop until his wife bleached the patient's underwear, a classic history.

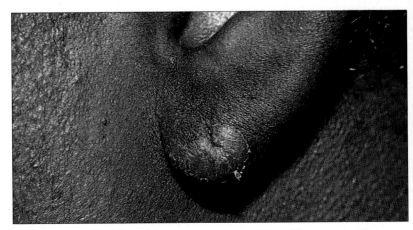

Figure 162. Nickel dermatitis from earrings. Nickel allergy is very common in women. The ear lobes become pruritic, inflamed and eczematous. Lichenification may result from chronic rubbing. Other areas in contact with nickel-containing metal may react. When told they have an allergy, patients often protest, saying they have used the item for years without trouble. This, however, is the typical story. It is only after years of exposure that the patient usually develops the allergy.

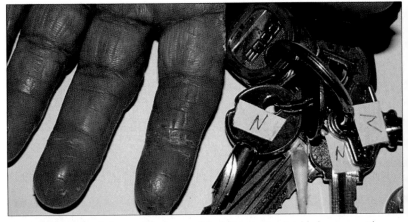

Figure 163. Hand dermatitis from nickel. The doctor should always consider allergic contact dermatitis in a patient presenting with an eczematous eruption. The hands are a common site for both allergic and irritant contact dermatitis because the hands come in contact with so many things. Patch testing in this patient showed a nickel allergy. Three of her keys tested positive to dimethylglioxime (a method to determine if an item contains nickel). Changing keys greatly improved the eruption.

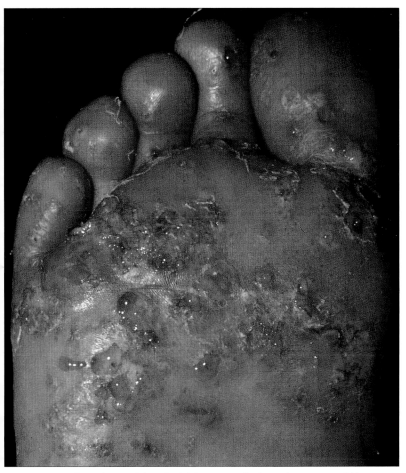

Figure 164. Shoe dermatitis mimicking pompholyx. This 10-year-old boy was treated for several years with the diagnosis of 'severe pompholyx'. It was only when patch testing was performed that an allergy to mercaptobenzathiozole was found. Rubber-free shoes cleared the feet completely!

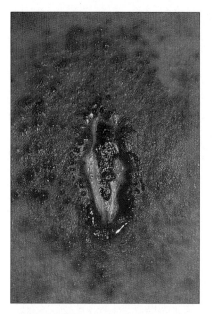

Figure 165. Bacitracin allergy. This patient developed redness, inflammation and dehiscence 10 days after a minor surgical excision. Allergic contact dermatitis to bacitracin was the cause. Always consider an allergy when the patient returns with a 'wound infection'.

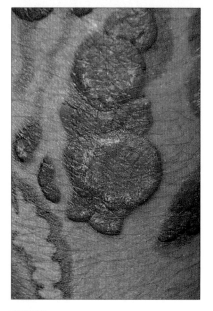

Figure 166. Tattoo allergy. Rarely a patient will be allergic to the tattoo pigment. Reaction to the red pigment, cinnabar (mercuric sulphide), is most common.

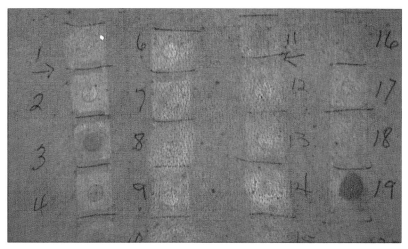

Figure 167. Patch testing, standard tray. When cutaneous allergy is suspected, patch testing should be done. Patches containing a standard tray of allergens are applied to the back for 48 hours. In this case, allergens 3 and 19 reacted.

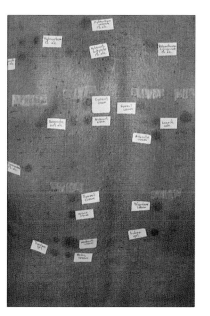

Figure 168. Patch testing, topical steroids. Patch testing beyond the standard tray is often necessary. All of the compounds being tested here are topical steroids. This patient reacted to over 20! Extended patch testing may be done in a variety of categories including fragrances, metals, preservatives, etc.

Black Dermatoses

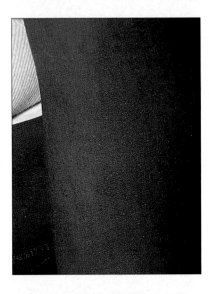

Figure 169. Futcher's lines. A sharp demarcation between the outer darker and the inner lighter skin on the arm of a black patient is characteristic. It represents a congenital difference in the darkness of pigment and one theory suggests that the dorsal skin is more heavily pigmented to provide better protection from the sun. Such a difference may become more obvious during pregnancy.

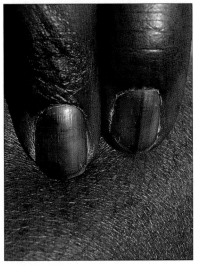

Figure 170. Longitudinal melanonychia. A longitudinal, pigmented streak of the nail commonly occurs in black patients and is usually benign. (See also **Figure 419**.)

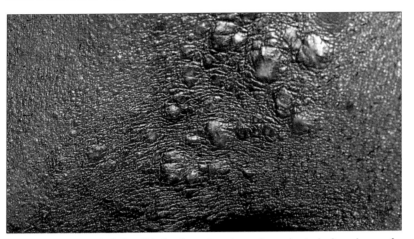

Figure 171. Pseudofolliculitis barbae. Papules and pustules in the beard area of a Black patient who tries for a close shave is characteristic. The curly whiskers curl into the skin, causing swelling and inflammation. Shaving often cuts or traumatizes these papules, adding to the problem.

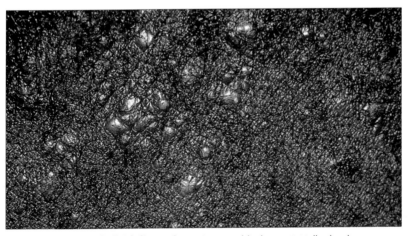

Figure 172. Acne keloidalis nuchae. A young black man initially develops a follicular, pustular eruption on the nape of the neck. Shaving the head and wearing a collar may precipitate the condition. Keloidal formation is signaled by the development of firm, follicular papules. The coexistence of pseudofolliculitis barbae has been noted in many patients.

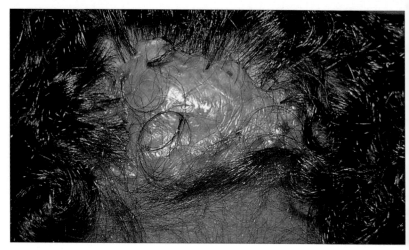

Figure 173. Acne keloidalis nuchae. Large keloids may form as well as polytrichia (tufts of hair emanating from the same opening), sinus tracts, pus and scarring alopecia.

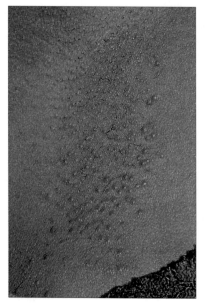

Figure 174. Fox–Fordyce disease. Uniformly distributed, pruritic, flesh-colored papules in the axilla, areola, groin and perineum are characteristic. Women at puberty or later are typically affected with men developing lesions only one-tenth as often.

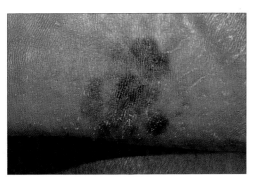

Figure 175. Acral melanoma. Melanoma in dark-skinned patients is rare but when it does occur, the palms, soles and nails are preferred locations. This lesion on the sole had grown slowly over several years.

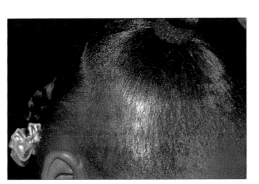

Figure 176. Traction alopecia. Extensive hair loss may occur in young Black girls who wear tight pony tails or braids. Inflammation is usually not seen, although follicular pustules may occasionally occur.

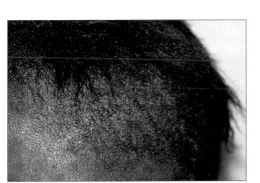

Figure 177. Hair damage causing hair loss. Significant hair damage and subsequent loss may be caused by the chemicals used to treat the hair. Excessive brushing may also be contributory.

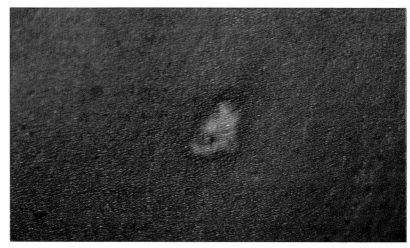

Figure 178. Post-cryotherapy hypopigmentation. Cryotherapy should always be used with caution in a dark-skinned patient, as a white spot may result. This patient had her axillary tags frozen.

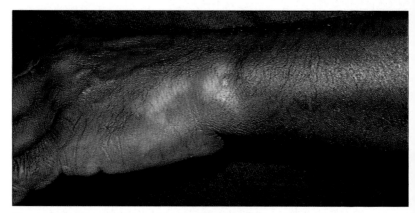

Figure 179. Steroid-induced hypopigmentation. Dark-skinned patients may develop localized hypopigmentation from either the application of a high potency topical steroid or from intralesional corticosteroid injection (as was done in this case into the wrist joint).

For related diseases, see also follicular eczema (**Figure 47**) and dermatosis papulosa nigra (**Figure 405**).

Bullous Disorders

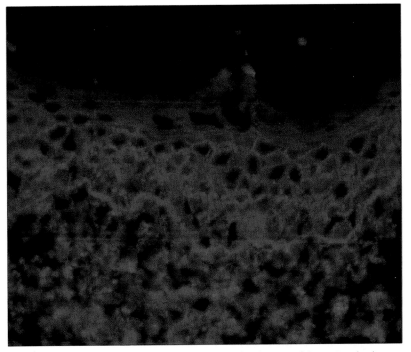

Figure 180. Immunofluorescence, paraneoplastic pemphigus. Rarely, the body's own immune system attacks the skin, causing weakness and subsequent bulla formation. The target antigen determines the level of separation, the distribution of lesions and, thus, the clinical findings. Immunofluorescence performed on a biopsy specimen (direct immunofluorescence) or from serum applied to a tissue substrate (indirect immunofluorescence) is invaluable in diagnosing and categorizing this class of diseases. The figure here shows both intercellular and basement membrane zone (BMZ) binding of IgG in paraneoplastic pemphigus. (Courtesy of WP Daniel Su, MD., from *Journal of the American Academy of Dermatology*, 1994; **30**, 841–844.)

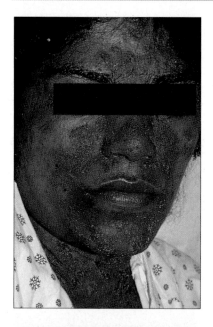

Figure 181. Pemphigus foliaceus.
Erosions, bulla and crusted plaques affecting the face, chest and elsewhere occur in pemphigus foliaceus. Some patients may have their disease exacerbated by UV-light exposure. The separation is in the upper epidermis and DIF shows intercellular IgG and/or C3. An endemic type also known as fogo selvagem occurs primarily in Brazil and mainly affects children and young adults.

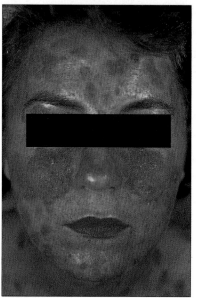

Figure 182. Pemphigus erythematosus. Also known as Senear–Usher syndrome, this variant of pemphigus presents with red, scaly, erosive, bullous or hyperkeratotic lesions on the nose and cheeks—an appearance and distribution similar to lupus erythematosus. Sunlight may aggravate the condition. DIF shows IgG and/or C3 intercellularly as well as along the BMZ. IIF is usually positive. A low positive antinuclear antibody may be present in approximately 30% of patients. (Courtesy of James Steger, MD.)

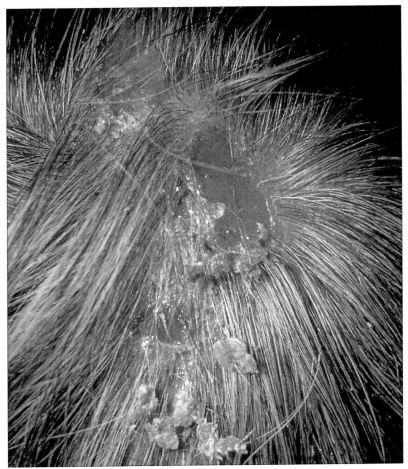

Figure 183. Pemphigus vulgaris, erosions, scalp. Widespread, flaccid bullae and crusted erosions are shown in a middle-aged patient with pemphigus vulgaris. The separation is intraepidermal and DIF shows intercellular IgG and/or C3. IIF is usually positive and its titer may correlate with disease activity. Untreated pemphigus vulgaris has a high mortality rate. (Courtesy of Bob Butler, MD.)

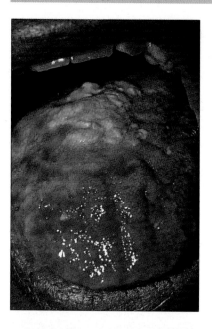

Figure 184. Pemphigus vulgaris, tongue. Oral erosions are very common in pemphigus vulgaris. Indeed, the patient may present with only oral ulcerations. Eating may be impaired.

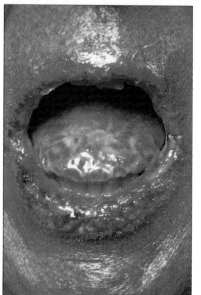

Figure 185. Paraneoplastic pemphigus, oral cavity. This recently recognized entity resembles pemphigus but is usually associated with a neoplasm. Extensive erosions of the oral cavity, conjunctiva, vagina and lips are characteristic. The mucosal erosions frequently extend beyond the vermilion border of the lips, as illustrated here. Average age of onset is 60 years. Associated neoplasms include bronchogenic squamous cell carcinoma, non-Hodgkin's lymphoma and chronic lymphocytic leukemia among others. Mortality is high. (Courtesy of WP Daniel Su, MD., and reproduced with permission from *Journal of the American Academy of Dermatology*, 1994; **30**, 841–844.)

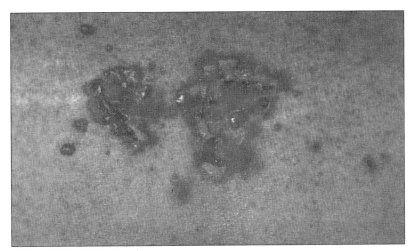

Figure 186. Paraneoplastic pemphigus. Cutaneous lesions do occur and may resemble pemphigus vulgaris (as shown here), erythema multiforme, lichen planus or bullous pemphigoid. (Courtesy of WP Daniel Su, MD., and reproduced with permission from *Journal of the American Academy of Dermatology*, 1994; **30**, 841–844.)

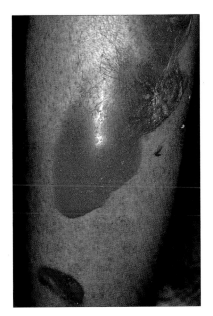

Figure 187. Bullous pemphigoid.
Large, tense, thick-walled bullae occur in bullous pemphigoid. Oral involvement is less common than in pemphigus vulgaris. The separation is subepidermal and direct immunofluorescence shows IgG and/or C3 along the BMZ. (Courtesy of Department of Dermatology, UCSD.)

Figure 188. Bullous pemphigoid, urticarial plaques, back. Occasionally, bullous pemphigoid may present only with fixed, pruritic, urticarial plaques in an older adult.

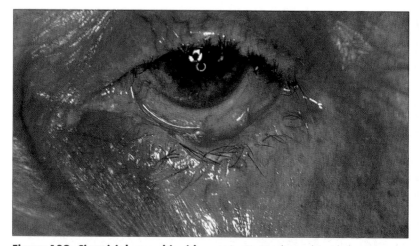

Figure 189. Cicatricial pemphigoid, eye. In cicatricial pemphigoid, the eye may be affected by a chronic conjunctivitis, burning and excessive tearing. Later, conjunctival shrinkage, entropion, corneal opacities and trichiasis may occur. If untreated, fibrous adhesions may attach both lids to the eye and ultimately blindness can develop. The level of separation is subepidermal and direct immunofluorescence shows IgG and/or C3 at the BMZ. IIF may be positive. (Courtesy of Eliot Mostow, MD.)

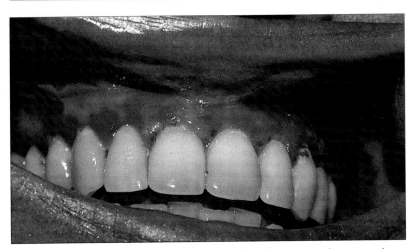

Figure 190. Cicatricial pemphigoid, gums. The oral mucosa is also commonly involved, causing oral ulceration and/or a desquamating gingivitis, as pictured here. The nasal, pharyngeal, laryngeal, esophageal and/or anogenital regions may be affected as well.

Figure 191. Cicatricial pemphigoid, Brunsting–Perry type. The skin may be affected in cicatricial pemphigoid in 10–25% of patients. The most common pattern is a localized form where recurrent blisters of the head and neck heal with scarring. This form has been termed Brunsting–Perry pemphigoid. This picture of an older man's forehead shows a flaccid bulla in the upper left and an erosion in the lower right.

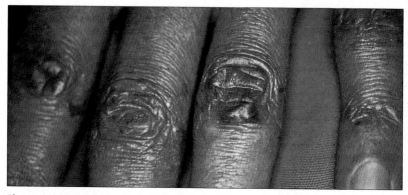

Figure 192. Epidermolysis bullosa acquisita. Trauma-induced bullae, milia and atrophic scars symmetric on the dorsa of the hands, feet and elbows occur in epidermolysis bullosa acquisita. The disease may be confused clinically with bullous pemphigoid or porphyria cutanea tarda. The separation is subepidermal and the patient's serum characteristically reacts to the dermal side of salt-split skin. (Courtesy of Eliot Mostow, MD.)

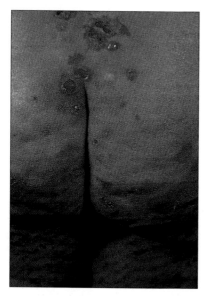

Figure 193. Dermatitis herpetiformis. A chronic, intensely pruritic vesicular rash that affects the knees, sacrum, back, posterior axillary folds and the elbows symmetrically is characteristic of dermatitis herpetiformis. Vesicles may not be found as the patient may scratch them away. The separation is subepidermal and DIF is usually positive for IgA in the dermal papillae. Gluten, the presumed causative antigen, is a protein found in most cereals, except rice and corn. A gluten-sensitive enteropathy is present and most patients have villous atrophy, although most do not have diarrhea. (Courtesy of James Steger, MD.)

Connective Tissue Disorders

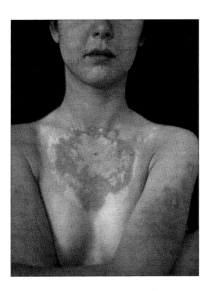

Figure 194. Systemic lupus erythematosus, butterfly rash.
Bilateral erythema of the cheeks and malar eminences (butterfly rash) or a more extensive photodistributed rash may be seen in systemic lupus erythematosus (SLE). Antinuclear antibody is usually positive—often with a positive anti-double-stranded DNA. Other findings include discoid rash, oral ulcers, photosensitivity, renal disease, neurologic disease, arthritis, serositis, hematologic disorders or immunologic disorders. (Courtesy of James Steger, MD.)

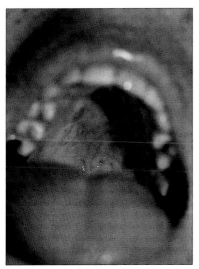

Figure 195. Systemic lupus erythematosus, oral ulceration.
Oral ulcerations may occur in both systemic and discoid lupus erythematosus (DLE).

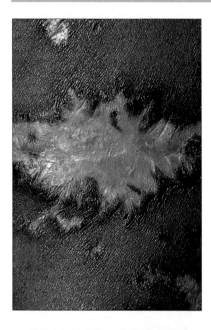

Figure 196. Discoid lupus erythematosus. Erythematous, hypopigmented, atrophic lesions occurring in photoexposed areas are typical of discoid lesions of chronic cutaneous lupus erythematosus. The border is often hyperpigmented, as illustrated here, and significant scarring may occur.

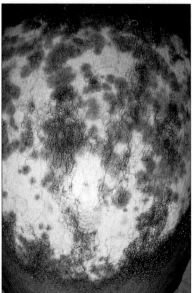

Figure 197. Discoid lupus erythematosus, alopecia. Significant scarring alopecia may occur in DLE. (Courtesy of Michael O Murphy, MD.)

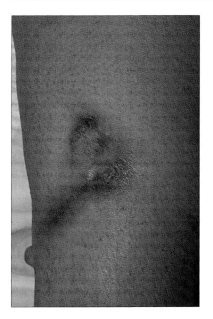

Figure 198. Lupus profundus.
Involvement of the underlying fat by lupus erythematosus may cause lipoatrophy and significant depression. Involvement of the upper, outer arm is a characteristic site. The overlying skin may be relatively unaffected or show changes typical of DLE.

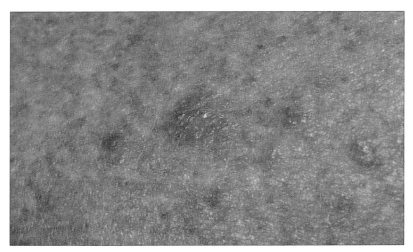

Figure 199. Subacute cutaneous lupus erythematosus, psoriasiform lesions. In this variant of lupus erythematosus, two cutaneous forms occur. Red, scaly papules and plaques in the photoexposed areas (here on the upper back) may occur.

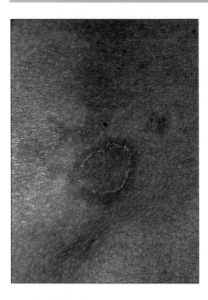

Figure 200. Subacute cutaneous lupus erythematosus, annular lesions. Alternatively, annular, red, scaly lesions may affect the trunk, especially the back, but also the arms and hands. Severe renal or CNS disease usually does not occur in subacute cutaneous lupus erythematosus. SS-A (Ro) antibodies are commonly found.

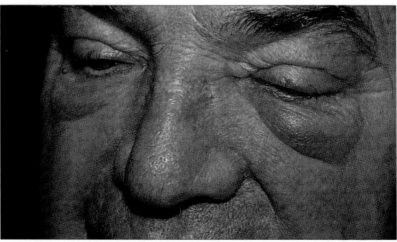

Figure 201. Dermatomyositis, periorbital edema. Periorbital edema with a violaceous hue is classic of dermatomyositis. A photodistributed eruption may be seen on the chest, upper back and arms (See **Figure 438**). Proximal muscle weakness is the classic systemic sign. There is a subset of patients with skin disease but without muscle involvement. There is a 15% incidence of cancer in adults but not for children (see **Figure 114**) under 16 years of age.

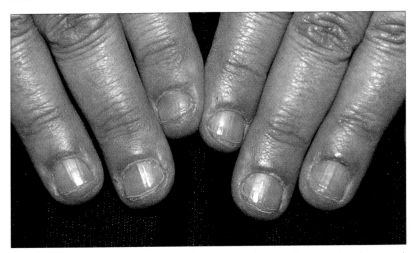

Figure 202. Dermatomyositis, periungual erythema. Periungual erythema and telangiectasias occur.

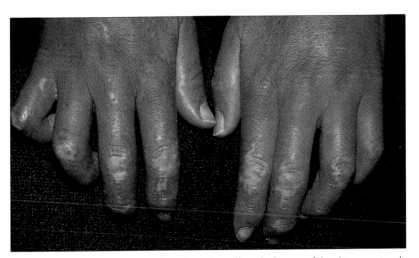

Figure 203. Scleroderma, sclerodactyly. Diffuse thickening of the skin associated with Raynaud's phenomenon, pulmonary, esophogeal and/or cardiac involvement is characteristic of scleroderma, also known as systemic sclerosis. The term sclerodactyly refers to induration of the digits, and is illustrated here. The patient has extended her fingers as much as possible. Note the erythema and depigmentation over the digits. Ulceration of the fingertips and over the knuckles occurs and can be debilitating.

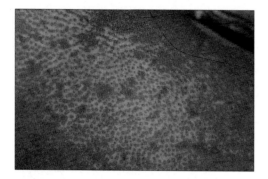

Figure 204. Scleroderma, polka-dot pattern. When depigmentation occurs in scleroderma, the perifollicular region is often spared, resulting in a polka-dot pattern as shown here. Note the similarity to repigmenting vitiligo (**Figure 469**).

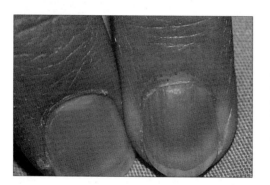

Figure 205. Scleroderma, nailfold capillaries. Dilated and distorted capillary loops alternating with avascular areas occur in systemic sclerosis and dermatomyositis. Nailfold bleeding may occur. In this illustration, the finger on the left is normal.

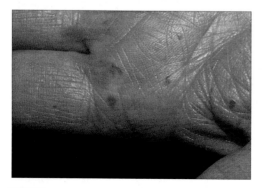

Figure 206. CREST syndrome, telangiectatic mats. **C**alcinosis cutis, **R**aynaud's phenomenon, **e**sophogeal dysfunction, **s**clerodactyly and **t**elangiectasias comprise the CREST syndrome, a variant of systemic scleroderma. Anticentromere antibodies are most characteristic of CREST but may also be found in systemic scleroderma patients.

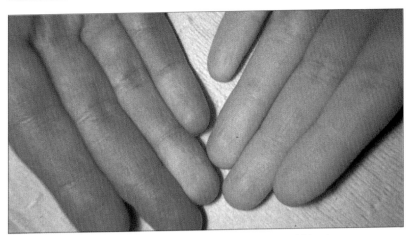

Figure 207. Raynaud's phenomenon. Sharply demarcated blanching occurs initially, followed by cyanosis and subsequently hyperemia in Raynaud's phenomenon. One or multiple fingers may be affected and cold exposure is the classic precipitating factor. Associations include collagen vascular disease, certain drugs and arterial disease (e.g. thromboangiitis obliterans). When idiopathic, the term Raynaud's disease is used. (Courtesy of James Rasmussen, MD.)

Figure 208. Morphea. The center is ivory white with a border of erythema. The skin is indurated on palpation. Women are more commonly affected and multiple lesions may occur. Very rarely, patients may go on to develop systemic sclerosis. Morphea and lichen sclerosis may coexist.

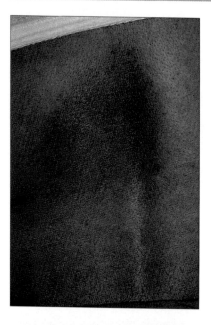

Figure 209. Atrophoderma of Pasini and Pierini. Tan-to-light-brown atrophic patches varying in size from several centimeters to tens of centimeters on the back of a young woman are characteristic. This disease is closely related to, and at times may resemble, morphea. The darker color of the lesions compared with the skin adds to their appearance of being depressed. However, the lesions are atrophic and the dermal atrophy of some of the lesions is so pronounced that a distinct 'drop off' at the edge is palpable.

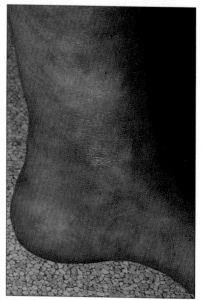

Figure 210. Linear scleroderma. A band-like linear induration, often with hypo- or hyperpigmented areas is characteristic. A deep component with fixation to underlying structures may be present. Joint pains are common and joint contractures caused by skin and tissue involvement may occur. Antinuclear antibody may be strongly positive. This woman's lesion extended the length of her inner leg.

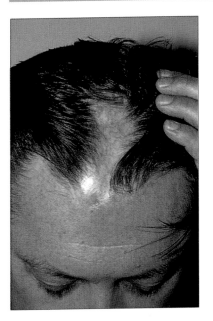

Figure 211. En coup de sabre. A linear, indurated depression running vertically just to one side of the midline on the face is characteristic of en coup de sabre, a variant of morphea. The lesion may extend to the scalp causing an alopetic streak as shown here, or it may spread downward to involve the nose, lips and chin.

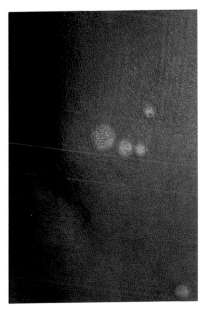

Figure 212. Lichen sclerosis, skin. These ivory white papules and plaques may occur anywhere on the skin, although the trunk is the preferred site. Note the characteristic follicular plugging. This young girl's lesions occurred on the ankles.

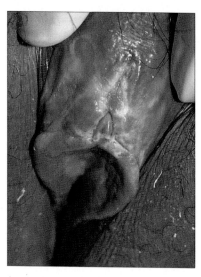

Figure 213. Lichen sclerosis, vulva.
Vulvar lichen sclerosis develops symmetrically about the vagina and rectum and tends to affect either prepubescent girls or perimenopausal women. Pruritus, burning pain, dyspareunia, dysuria, vaginal discharge, anal or genital bleeding, labial stenosis or fusion, constipation (especially in children), erosion, contraction and squamous cell carcinoma may occur.

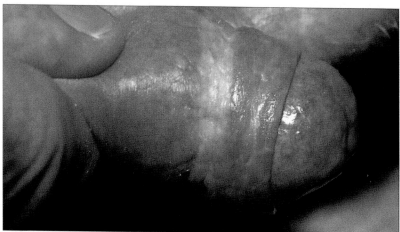

Figure 214. Balanitis xerotica obliterans. The glans and/or foreskin become white, smooth and atrophic in lichen sclerosis of the penis, which is also called balanitis xerotica obliterans. Erosions, hemorrhage, decreased sensation of the glans, painful erections and scarring with phimosis may occur. This disease represents a common cause of phimosis in boys. Squamous cell carcinoma may rarely occur.

For related diseases, see also pemphigus erythematosus (**Figure 182**).

Drug-Related Disorders

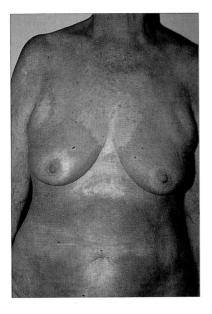

Figures 215 and 216.
Maculopapular drug eruption.
Erythematous macules and smooth papules scattered symmetrically across the trunk and elsewhere are characteristic. When faced with a patient on multiple medications, a book that lists specific drugs, the characteristic reaction pattern and the likelihood of such an eruption, is invaluable.

Figure 216.

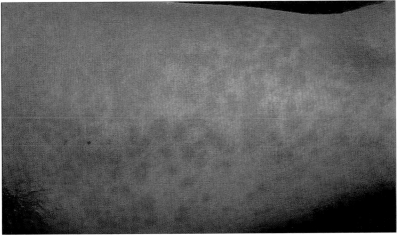

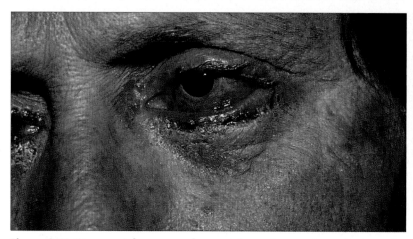

Figure 217. Stevens–Johnson syndrome. Inflammation, crusting and redness of the conjunctival, oral and genital mucosa develop acutely. Headache, fever and malaise also occur. Inability to eat, fluid loss, and infection are significant complications. Drugs are the most common cause (e.g. penicillins, phenytoin, sulfonamides) but an infection may be implicated.

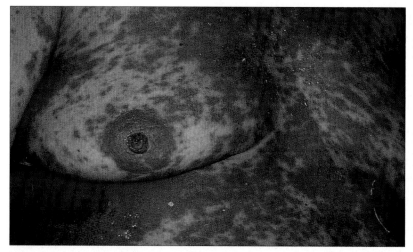

Figure 218. Stevens–Johnson syndrome. The rash of Stevens–Johnson syndrome may resemble the classic maculopapular drug rash but is often more dusky red, with areas of necrosis. Erosions, as illustrated below this woman's right breast, commonly occur.

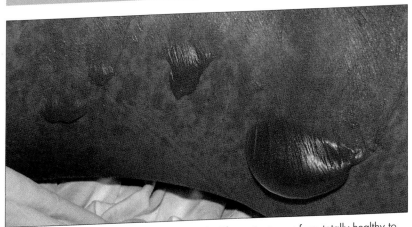

Figure 219. Toxic epidermal necrolysis. The patient goes from totally healthy to life-threateningly ill within a few days. A prodrome of malaise and fever is followed by diffuse erythema and edema of the skin. Bullae then develop, which enlarge until the epidermis sloughs off in large sheets. Mortality is between 25 and 50%. Any drug may be implicated but the most common are sulfonamides, non-steroidal anti-inflammatories and anticonvulsants.

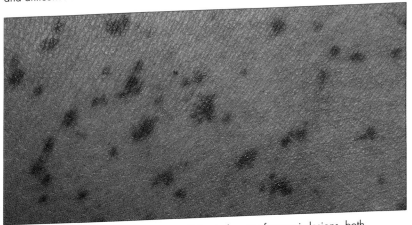

Figure 220. Hypersensitivity vasculitis. A shower of purpuric lesions, both palpable and non-palpable, concentrated on the legs occurs in hypersensitivity vasculitis. Associated symptoms include fever, malaise, nausea and arthralgias. Often, this eruption resolves before a work-up can be completed. The most common cause is a drug, but many systemic diseases have been implicated including inflammatory bowel disease, large vessel vasculitis, malignancy, infection, cryoglobulins and collagen vascular disease.

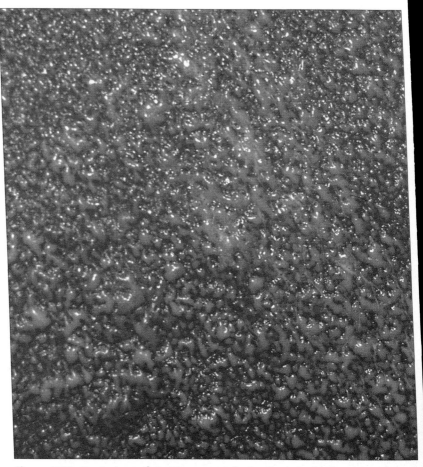

Figure 221. Acute exanthematous pustulosis. A rapidly developing non-follicular pustular eruption on diffusely erythematous skin is characteristic of acute exanthematous pustulosis, also called toxic pustuloderma. The onset is typically within a day of exposure to the offending agent, which in most cases is a drug. The pustules are sterile.

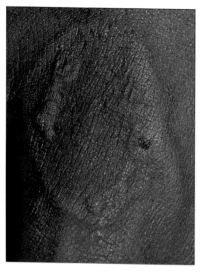

Figure 222. Fixed drug eruption, solitary. Single or multiple, dusky-red, round or oval lesions occurring repeatedly in a fixed site after each exposure to the offending drug are characteristic. Crusting or blistering, as shown here, may occur. Typical drugs to consider include tetracycline, sulfa drugs, ampicillin and phenolphthalein.

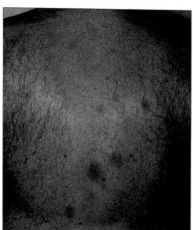

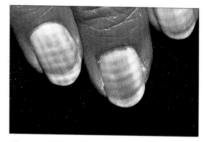

Figure 224. Chemotherapy. Transverse white lines that grow out with the nail may occur in association with chemotherapy—analogous to Beau's lines (**Figure 425**).

Figure 223. Fixed drug eruption, multiple. With each subsequent exposure to the drug, the initial lesion may increase in size and additional lesions may develop. This patient noticed an ever increasing number of lesions with each episode. Phenolphthalein in a laxative was the cause.

For related diseases, see also doxycycline (**Figure 148**), tetracycline (**Figure 149**), minocycline (**Figures 150 and 151**), and photodrug eruption (**Figure 434**).

Eczematous Dermatoses

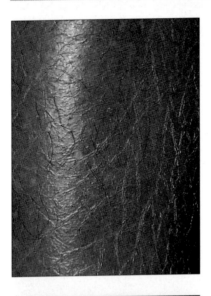

Figure 225. Xerosis, legs. The skin may be thought of as a wet sponge covered by a thin oil membrane. When the surface oil is depleted, the sponge dries out. An atopic background, dry, cold weather, frequent water contact, advanced age and irritants predispose to dry skin, also known as xerosis. The shins are commonly affected.

Figure 226. Asteatotic eczema, legs. When the skin's superficial water barrier is lost, the underlying skin dries out and may become inflamed. The legs of elderly people in the winter months are commonly affected. The skin appears erythematous and cracked with wide but superficial fissures.

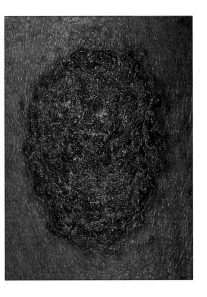

Figure 227. Nummular eczema.
The appearance of this lesion is **not** that of ringworm (**Figure 298**). The redness and inflammation is uniformly distributed throughout. An 'active border' is not seen. As was typical in this patient, multiple lesions tend to erupt on the arms and legs. Pruritis is usually significant. Risk factors include excessive bathing (e.g. more than 10 minutes), other prolonged water exposure (e.g. regular swimming) and dry, cold air.

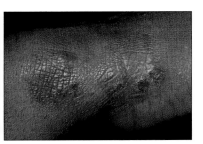

Figure 228. Lichen simplex chronicus.
Scratching is never good. It opens the skin up to infection, prevents healing and may induce lesions through Koebnerization. It also hides characteristic changes of any primary lesion making the doctor's work that much harder. Illustrated here are two chronic, lichenified, excoriated plaques in a patient with atopic dermatitis. Accentuation of the skin lines (lichenification) is seen.

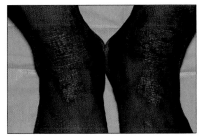

Figure 229. Lichen simplex chronicus.
Lichen simplex chronicus may occur virtually anywhere but common sites include the ankle, shin, scrotum, vulva, nape and side of the neck. It is often less threatening and more helpful when trying to elicit a history of chronic scratching to ask the patient, "Does it itch?" rather than asking, "Do you scratch?"

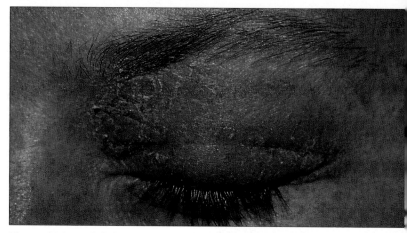

Figure 230. Eyelid dermatitis. Chronic redness and scaling about the eyes are very common, especially in women. The most common causes are allergic contact, irritant contact, atopic and seborrheic dermatitis. Work-up should include inquiry into the patient's occupation (e.g. any airborne matter, sawdust), use of potential allergens (e.g. nail polish, makeup, eyeliner, eye drops), a complete skin examination (to look for signs of atopic dermatitis, psoriasis or seborrheic dermatitis) and patch testing.

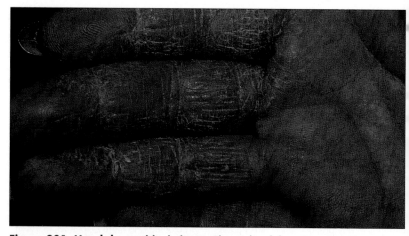

Figure 231. Hand dermatitis, irritant. Chronic hand dermatitis can pose a significant problem for the patient, doctor and employer. Inquiry should be made regarding the patient's occupation, hobbies, the frequency of hand washing and exposure to chemicals or irritants. Allergic contact dermatitis should be excluded. This woman developed an irritant hand dermatitis soon after having her first baby.

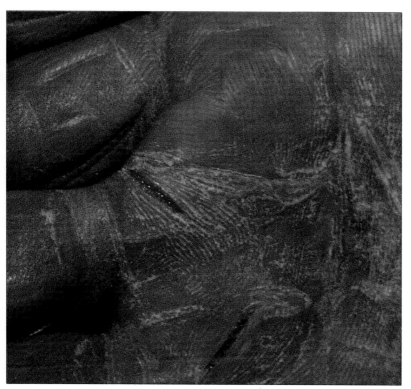

Figure 232. Hyperkeratotic eczema. Diffuse, thickened, fissured hyperkeratosis of the palms occurring in a middle-aged adult is characteristic. Patch testing and the potassium hydroxide examination to exclude other causes are important. Fissuring, as illustrated here, can be painful.

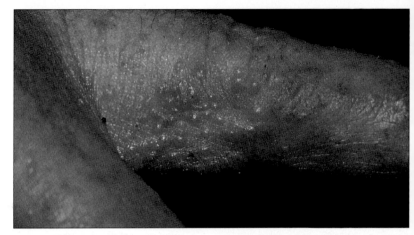

Figure 233. Pompholyx, vesicles. Tiny 'tapioca' vesicles of the sides of the fingers but also fingertips, palms and soles occur in this condition, also called dyshidrotic eczema. Areas may become red, scaly and weeping, and the patient usually complains of intense itching. A mild form may occur in which small vesicles rupture to form enlarging collarettes of scale. A severe form may occur with large palmar and plantar bullae.

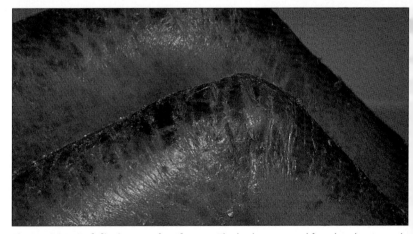

Figure 234. Exfoliative erythroderma. The body is covered from head to toe with erythema and variable scale. This presentation may be caused by various entities including a medication, psoriasis, atopic dermatitis, pityriasis rubra pilaris and most importantly cutaneous T-cell lymphoma. The initial work-up for patients who have no obvious cause includes a thorough history and physical exam, complex blood count and skin biopsy. If these are unrevealing, lymph node biopsy or CAT scan may be done.

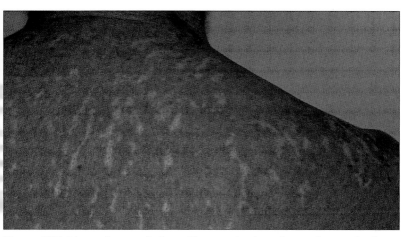

Figure 235. Neurotic excoriations. The upper back is a favorite location for the chronic picking and scratching that occurs in neurotic excoriations. Round-to-oval white scars accumulate over time. A primary dermatosis should be excluded as well as delusions of parasitosis.

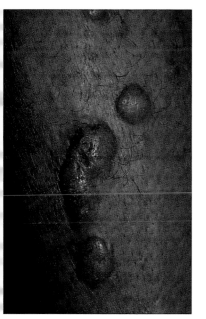

Figure 236. Prurigo nodularis.
Chronic scratching can eventually result in the formation of nodules.

Hair Disorders

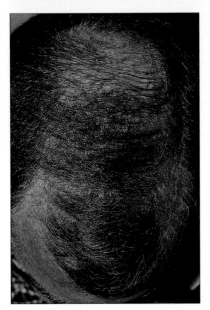

Figure 237. Androgenic alopecia, male. A young man in his 20s or 30s may become very distressed and seek medical help because of hair loss at the vertex and bilaterally along the frontotemporal areas. Individual hairs become smaller and the hairline recedes. Later, the forehead becomes taller and, finally, all terminal hair may be lost from the forehead to the vertex. Vertex baldness (but not frontal) has been associated with an increased risk for ischemic heart disease.

General work-up for hair loss in a woman. There is no figure for this legend because the majority of women who seek medical attention for thinning hair seem normal on examination. This is because a significant portion of the hair must be lost before the change is clinically apparent. The history and a physical and laboratory examination should exclude telogen effluvium, thyroid disease, hormonal abnormalities, drug-induced alopecia and low iron. If no cause is found, the diagnosis of androgenic alopecia is made.

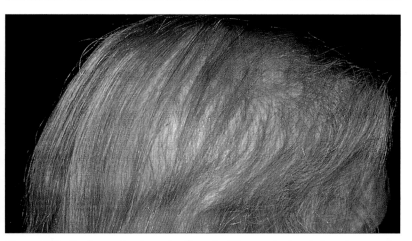

Figure 238. Androgenic alopecia, female. Women who lose hair as they age do so in a pattern different from men. The hairline is preserved but thinning develops from the frontal hairline to the vertex. A family history may or may not be found.

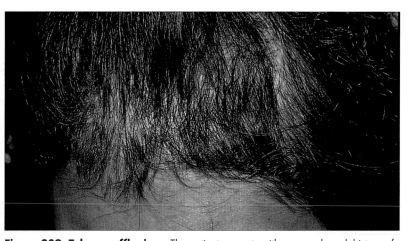

Figure 239. Telogen effluvium. The patient presents with a several week history of increased hair loss as seen on her pillow, brush or in the shower. She may pull at her hair in the office, showing how easily the hairs are removed. In this disease, hair loss occurs approximately 2–3 months after a stressful event. Causes include chronic systemic diseases (e.g. liver failure, renal failure, cancer), severe psychological stress, surgery and/or anesthesia, crash dieting, acute physical stress (e.g. high fever, severe bleeding) and giving birth.

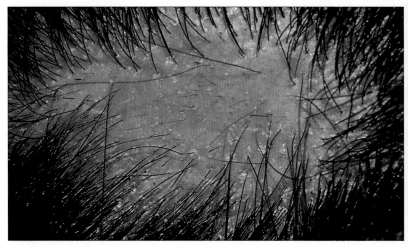

Figure 240. Alopecia areata, scalp. The sudden and near complete loss of hair in one or more circular patches is characteristic of alopecia areata, a disease that affects children and young adults preferentially. Short, blunt-ended hairs, tapered at the base (exclamation point hairs), may be seen near the margin of the alopecia.

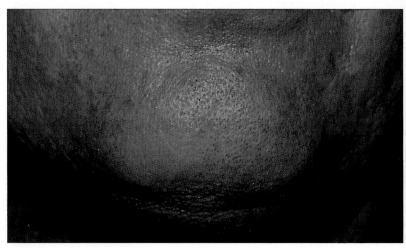

Figure 241. Alopecia areata, beard. The scalp is most commonly affected by alopecia areata but loss can occur in the eyebrows, eyelashes, beard and elsewhere.

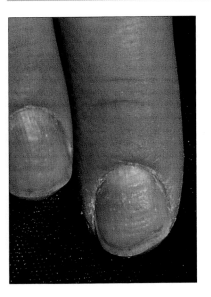

Figure 242. Alopecia areata, pits, nails. Pits may occur in the nail in a uniform grid-like pattern.

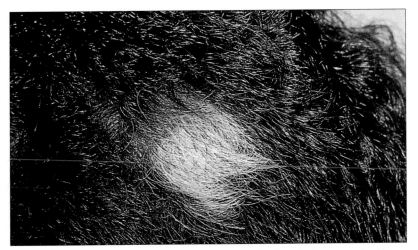

Figure 243. Alopecia areata, regrowth with all-white hair. Regrowth of hair occurs in most patients within the first year and in the vast majority within 2 years. The initial regrowing hair is usually normal color but may be white.

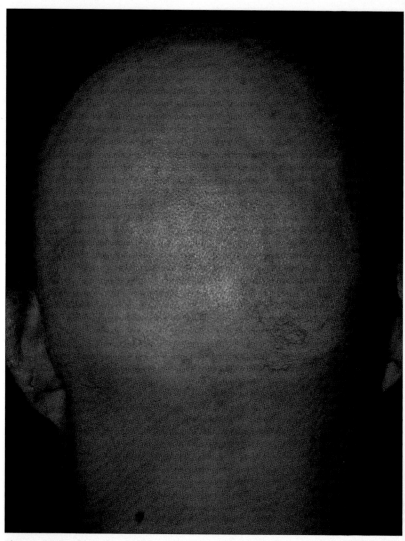

Figure 244. Alopecia totalis, scalp. When all of the scalp hair is lost in alopecia areata, the term alopecia totalis is used. When all hair everywhere is lost, the term alopecia universalis is used. The physician must be sensitive to the emotional and psychological distress that may accompany the loss of all one's hair. (Erythema nuchae is also seen.)

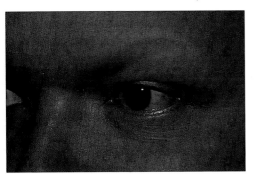

Figure 245. Alopecia universalis. Note the loss of both eyebrow hair and the eyelashes.

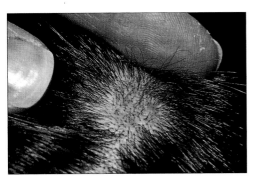

Figure 246. Trichotillomania, localized. Young girls may pull, twist or twirl their hair with such rapidity and force as to cause localized hair loss. One characteristic sign is that the remaining hairs are not uniform in length. The nails may be dystrophic from onychophagia but pits are not seen (as with alopecia areata).

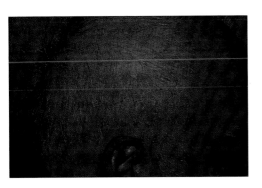

Figure 247. Anagen effluvium. A toxic insult to the body can preferentially affect the hair bulb due to its active metabolism. Diffuse hair loss can result. Cancer chemotherapeutic drugs are the most common offenders. Permanent damage is not done and hair regrowth is expected if the insult is removed.

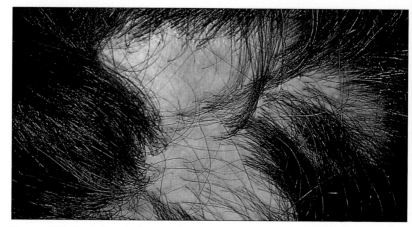

Figure 248. Pseudopelade. Round-to-oval, non-inflamed, white, alopetic areas of the scalp, like 'footprints in the snow' are characteristic. There may be perifollicular erythema early and moderate atrophy in late stages but no crust, scale or follicular hyperkeratosis is seen. Most patients are women. The course is chronic with slow progression. The key differential diagnoses are cutaneous lupus erythematosus and lichen planopilaris.

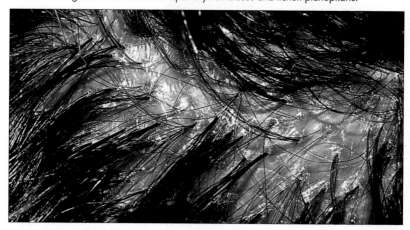

Figure 249. Tufted folliculitis. Tufted hairs or polytrichia forming in the setting of chronic *Staphylococcus aureus* infection of the scalp, acne keloidalis nuchae, folliculitis decalvans or dissecting cellulitis of the scalp are characteristic. This disease is not a single entity but a clinical finding in the setting of various inflammatory alopecias. The tufts of hair probably form through compaction by scars and inflammation.

See also discoid lupus erythematosus (**Figure 197**) and tinea capitis (**Figures 90–93**).

HIV-Related Dermatoses

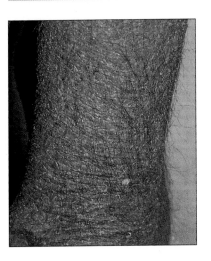

Figure 250. Xerosis/atopic diathesis. HIV-positive patients may develop significant xerosis (dry skin) and even an atopic diathesis.

Figure 251. Kaposi's sarcoma. HIV-related Kaposi's sarcoma (KS) usually presents as an asymptomatic, erythematous macule that later becomes raised and violaceous. Larger truncal lesions tend to be ovoid, following lines of cleavage as illustrated here. This angiomatous proliferation appears to be related to an infectious cofactor. Herpes DNA has been found in a high percentage of tissue specimens.

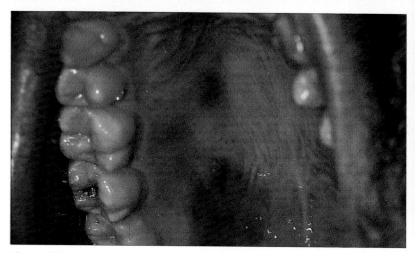

Figure 252. Kaposi's sarcoma, palate. KS lesions are common on the trunk, extremities and oral cavity (where the palate is preferred).

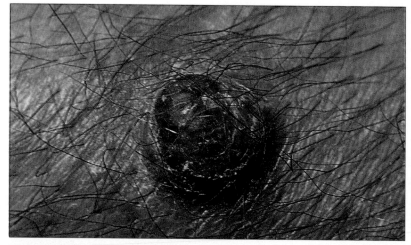

Figure 253. Bacillary angiomatosis. Pyogenic granuloma-like lesions, reddish-purple papulonodules and/or subcutaneous nodules in a patient with AIDS are characteristic. Systemic symptoms (e.g. fever, chills, malaise) as well as systemic involvement (especially of the liver) may occur. This disease represents an angiomatous proliferation caused by a bacteria (either *Bartonella hensela* or *B. quintana*) that is acquired most commonly from a cat bite, scratch or lick or possibly from cat fleas. (Courtesy of Caroline Thornton, MD.)

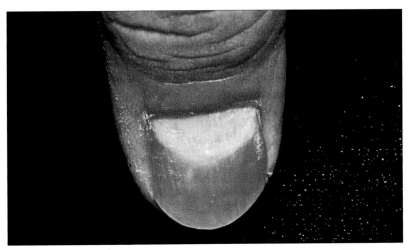

Figure 254. Proximal subungual onychomycosis. Hyperkeratotic debris accumulates on the undersurface in the most proximal portion of the nail plate. *Trichophyton rubrum* is the most common organism.

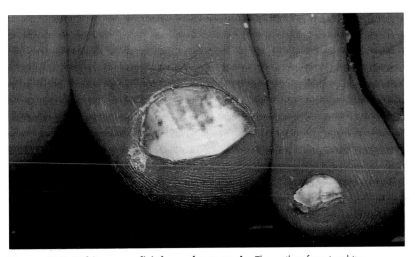

Figure 255. White superficial onychomycosis. The nail surface is white, keratotic and powdery in white superficial onychomycosis. The organism is usually *T. mentagrophites*. This condition also commonly occurs in immune competent patients.

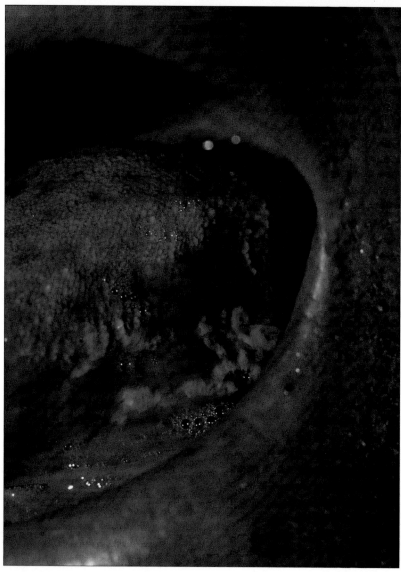

Figure 256. Oral hairy leukoplakia. White, verrucous, corrugated plaques on the sides of the tongue in an HIV-positive patient are characteristic. The lesions are usually asymptomatic. The Epstein–Barr virus is implicated as the etiologic factor.

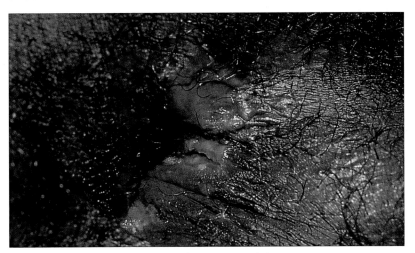

Figure 257. Perianal herpes simplex. A perianal ulcer in an HIV-positive patient represents a herpes simplex infection until proven otherwise.

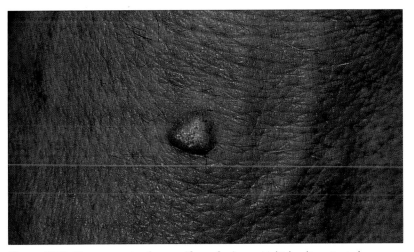

Figure 258. Herpes zoster/verruciform lesions. Multiple, disseminated hyperkeratotic, verrucous papules and plaques in an HIV-positive patient may represent chronic infection by the varicella zoster virus.

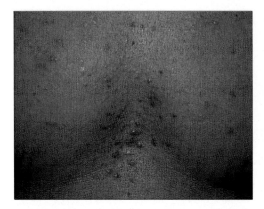

Figure 259. Eosinophilic folliculitis. Chronic pruritic, follicular papules of the trunk, neck and arms in an HIV-positive patient are characteristic. Occasionally, one can see a few intact pustules. Intense scratching often leads to bleeding, crusting and eroded papules. A bacterial folliculitis caused by *Staphylococcus* or *Pseudomonas* should be excluded.

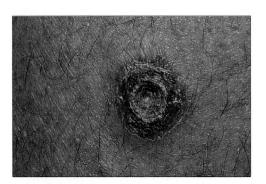

Figure 260. Psoriasis. A spectrum of diseases from psoriasis to manifestations of Reiter's syndrome may occur in HIV-positive patients. Psoriatic arthritis is more common in HIV-positive patients with psoriasis.

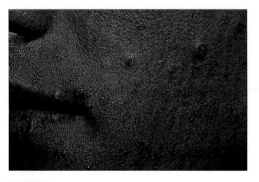

Figure 261. Molluscum contagiosum, beard. Innumerable flesh-colored papules of the beard are common in HIV-positive patients. Shaving may spread them throughout the beard area. The presence of organisms in clinically normal adjacent skin may explain its resistance to therapy.

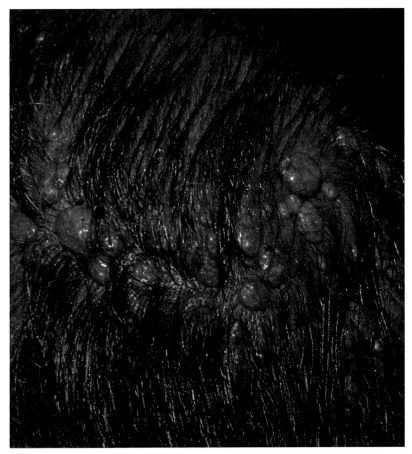

Figure 262. Molluscum contagiosum, giant. At times, the papules may become large presenting a difficult therapeutic problem.

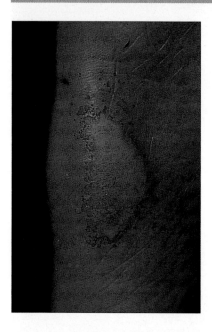

Figure 263. Pitted keratolysis.
Multiple 1–2 mm pits in a teenager wearing footwear for prolonged periods with sweating is typical. Causative bacteria include *Corynebacterium* and *Micrococcus sedentarius*.

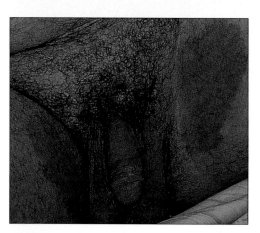

Figure 264. Erythrasma.
Corynebacterium minutissimum is the bacterium responsible for this mild, chronic superficial infection. Red-brown patches, commonly of the groin or axilla, with distinct borders and little to no scale occur.

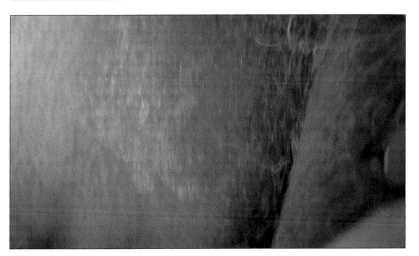

Figure 265. Erythrasma, coral red fluorescence. *C. minutissimum* creates a water-soluble porphyrin that fluoresces coral pink under Wood's light examination. This finding may be absent if the patient has recently bathed.

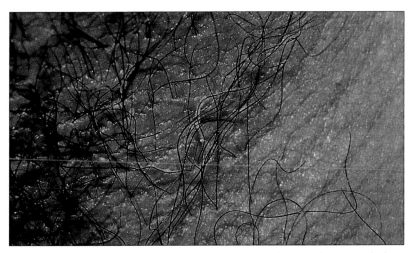

Figure 266. Trichomychosis axillaris. Yellow, red or black attachments on the hair representing bacterial colonization occurs in trichomycosis axillaris. *Corynebacterium tenuis* is one of the bacteria which has been identified.

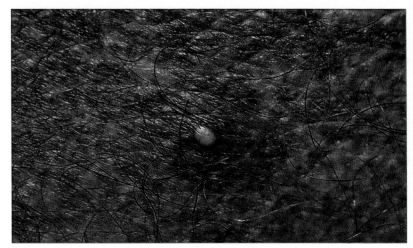

Figure 267. Staphylococcal folliculitis, pustule. Multiple follicular pustules scattered on the trunk may represent a bacterial folliculitis. Excoriations may mask the primary pustule. Culture establishes the diagnosis and can indicate the appropriate antibiotic choice.

Figure 268. Staphylococcal folliculitis, erythematous papules. Often, staphylococcal folliculitis lesions are deep-seated and appear only as erythematous papules.

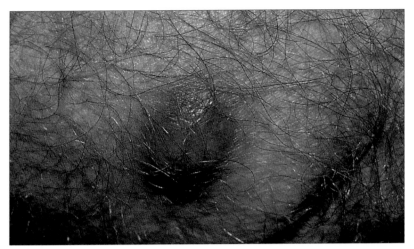

Figure 269. Furuncle. A furuncle or a boil begins as a tender, inflamed nodule that usually becomes fluctuant, points and ruptures.

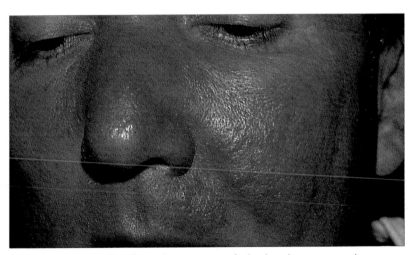

Figure 270. Erysipelas, face. The acute onset of a bright red, warm, spreading, edematous plaque on the cheek may represent a bacterial infection usually caused by *Streptococcus*. Fever or chills may accompany the rash and pustules or skin breakdown may occur.

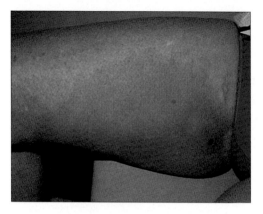

Figure 271. Erysipelas, leg. The acute onset of a warm, erythematous, edematous plaque that each day enlarges several to many centimeters is characteristic. Fever and chills or more severe skin changes (e.g. purpura, bullae, postbullous ulceration, necrosis, hypoesthesia or fluctuance) may suggest necrotizing fasciitis or pyomyositis. Risk factors include impaired venous or lymphatic return, diabetes mellitus, atherosclerosis, NSAID use and a pre-existing open lesion.

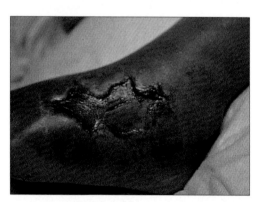

Figure 272. Necrotizing fasciitis. The so-called flesh eating bacteria—group A beta hemolytic *Streptococcus*—can cause significant tissue destruction rapidly. This 32-year-old woman developed pain, erythema and swelling of the foot followed by necrotic ulceration over a week. There was no history of trauma. (Courtesy of Roger Bitar, MD.)

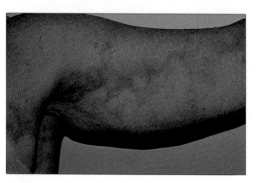

Figure 273. Lymphangitic streaking. This woman, postmastectomy, developed cellulitis of the forearm with subsequent lymphangitic streaking along the defective lymphatic system.

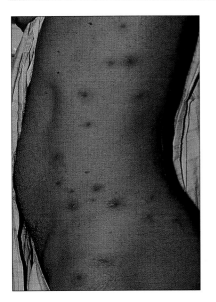

Figure 274. Hot-tub folliculitis. The typical patient with hot-tub folliculitis develops multiple pustules on top of urticarial bases scattered on the trunk and/or buttocks several days after using a hot tub contaminated by the Gram-negative bacterium *Pseudomonas aeruginosa*. Prolonged hydration and occlusion of the skin (e.g. by a tight bathing suit) promote infection.

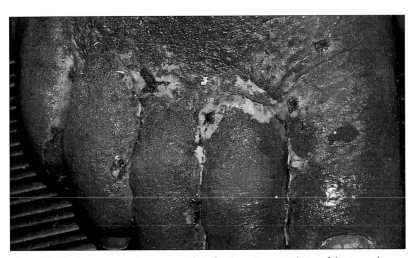

Figure 275. Gram-negative toe-web infection. Dermatophytes of the toe-web space may produce penicillin and streptomycin-like substances that allow Gram-negative bacteria to overgrow. The distal foot and toes become swollen, inflamed and malodorous. *Proteus* and *Pseudomonas* are often found. The affected patient often wears shoes most of the day.

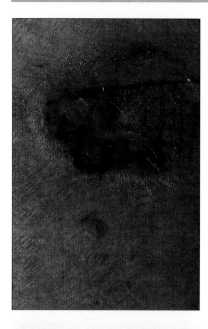

Figure 276. Ecthyma gangrenosum. One or multiple, well-defined areas of necrosis and ulceration may develop as a manifestation of *Pseudomonas aeruginosa* infection. The initial lesion is often a bulla or hemorrhagic pustule. The classic adult with ecthyma gangrenosum is a very ill, immunocompromised patient in the intensive care unit. Infants may be affected in the diaper area.

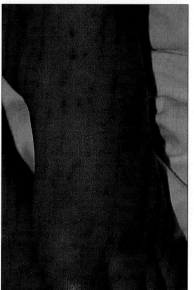

Figure 277. Neisseria meningitidis, distal purpura. The classic patient is a child or teenager who acutely develops severe headache, nausea, vomiting and fever. Meningeal symptoms may occur and the mental state may deteriorate to disorientation or even coma. Hypotensive shock and death may rapidly ensue. A petechial rash, often on the extensor hands, arms and feet is characteristic.

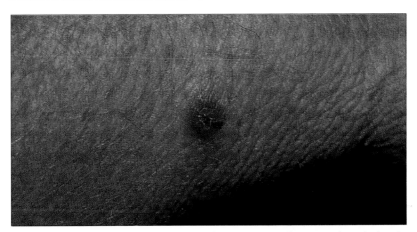

Figure 278. Cat scratch disease, papule at cat scratch. A scratch on the hand or arm by a cat followed weeks later by painful lymphadenopathy that may suppurate is characteristic. The causative organism appears to be *Bartonella henselae*. Patients are likely to have a kitten, been scratched, licked on the face, bitten by a kitten or to have a kitten with fleas.

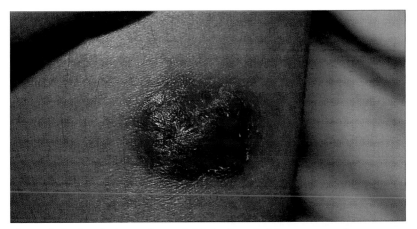

Figure 279. Atypical mycobacterial infection. A violaceous, crusted or hyperkeratotic papulonodule develops on the dorsal surface of the hand or finger, often over a knuckle. The disease is also known as a swimming pool or fish tank granuloma. If acquired from an aquarium, the dominant hand is typically affected. If acquired from a pool, any site of trauma may be affected. Any hobbies or occupations that bring the patient in contact with fish are predisposing factors. This granuloma is caused by an atypical mycobacterium, usually *Mycobacterium marinum*.

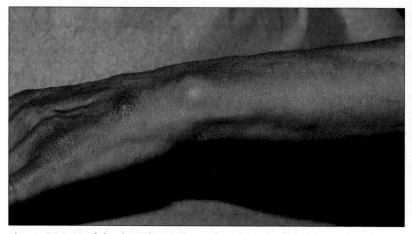

Figure 280. Nodular lymphangitis. Tender inflamed nodules, progressing up the arm originating from a traumatic injury on the hand—so-called sporotrichoid spread—are characteristic of nodular lymphangitis, also called lymphocutaneous syndrome. The most common atypical mycobacterium to spread in a sporotrichoid fashion is *Mycobacterium marinum,* as shown here. Other infectious agents that may be found include *Leishmania, Nocardia brasiliensis, Francisella tularensis* and, of course, *Sporothrix schenckii.*

Figure 281. Tuberculosis verrucosa cutis. A chronic, warty plaque on the hand, knees, ankles or buttocks (as shown here) is characteristic of this infection caused by *Mycobacterium tuberculosis.* Inoculation may have occurred from the patient's own saliva, another's saliva (e.g. sitting on spit) or from work (e.g. a pathologist with a prosector's wart).

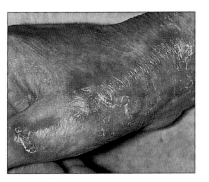

Figure 282. Lupus vulgaris. A hyperkeratotic, crusted, granulomatous plaque or plaques on the face or elsewhere is characteristic. An apple jelly color is seen on diascopy (pressure to remove the blood with a glass slide). This disease represents an infection by *Mycobacterium tuberculosis* in a patient with moderate to high immunity and may have developed from local inoculation, lymphatic or hematogenous spread. (Courtesy of Christopher EM Griffiths, MD.)

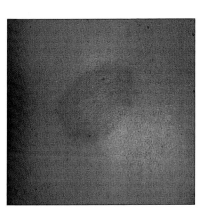

Figure 283. Erythema migrans. A red papule or macule which rapidly enlarges to form an annular lesion within a month of, and at the site of, a tick bite is characteristic. The primary lesion may also be an urticarial plaque without central clearing or have a central dusky purpuric or necrotic appearance. The infecting organism is *Borrelia bergdorferi*. (Courtesy of Daniel K Frum, MD.)

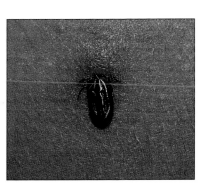

Figure 284. Tick bite by *Ixodes pacificus.* The vector for Lyme disease is the *Ixodes* tick. It appears that the tick must be attached for at least 24 hours to infect. Methods that help prevent Lyme disease include avoiding endemic, wooded areas, applying insect repellent, wearing long pants and long-sleeved shirts, tucking pants into socks and checking regularly for ticks, removing them promptly if found.

See also impetigo (**Figure 49**) and bullous impetigo (**Figure 124**).

Superficial Fungal Infections

Figure 285. Intertrigo. The skin of the infra-mammary fold may become red, scaly, moist or macerated. Obese women with large breasts exposed to hot humid climates are most commonly affected. Although intertrigo is not an infectious process, secondary infection commonly occurs.

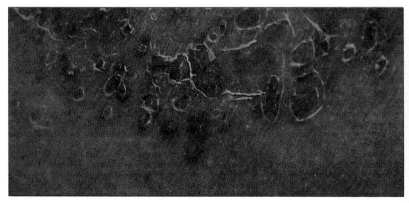

Figure 286. Candidiasis, satellite pustules. Intertrigo is often secondarily infected by candida. Satellite pustules are characteristic.

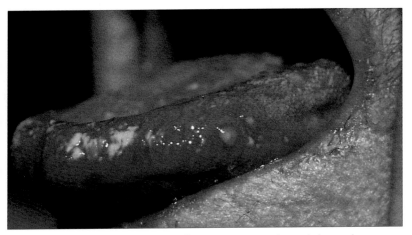

Figure 287. Thrush. In adults, HIV infection, corticosteroid use, diabetes, dentures, old age and any cause of depressed cell-mediated immunity are risk factors for candidiasis of the oral mucosa. White, creamy papules and plaques occur and the underlying mucosa may be red and inflamed. Healthy infants, especially those that are premature, and children on antibiotics may also be affected.

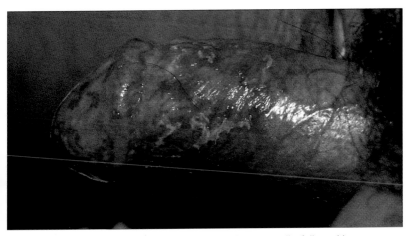

Figure 288. Candida balanitis. Bright red erythema initially, followed by minute pustules on the glans penis is characteristic. Uncircumcised men are at higher risk. A white, creamy coating may develop. The organism may have been obtained from the patient's own gastrointestinal tract or a sexual partner's vagina. In severe cases, dysuria, pain with intercourse and phimosis may occur.

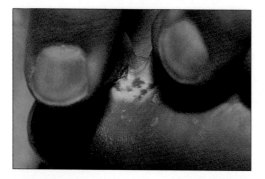

Figure 289. Tinea pedis, interdigital. Relatively asymptomatic, uncomplicated scaling of the web space is characteristic of simple dermatophyte infection. The web between the 4th and 5th toes is most often affected. When a mixed infection of dermatophyte and bacteria develops, the area may become white, macerated and malodorous.

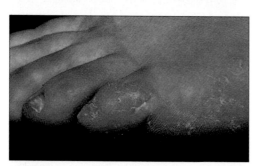

Figure 290. Tinea pedis. Redness and scaling of the web spaces initially but later over some or all of the sole (moccasin distribution) are characteristic. Potassium hydroxide examination or culture is confirmatory.

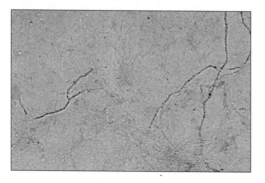

Figure 291. Potassium hydroxide examination. Virtually any relatively flat, scaly lesion should raise the suspicion of fungal infection. The potassium hydroxide examination is invaluable because of its ease, simplicity and quick results. Abundant scale is scraped onto a microscopic slide with a blade and covered with a coverslip. KOH 10–20% with or without dimethyl sulfoxide (DMSO) is added. Fungal hyphae stand out as linear, branching, septate filaments of uniform width. (Courtesy of Terence C. O'Grady, MD.)

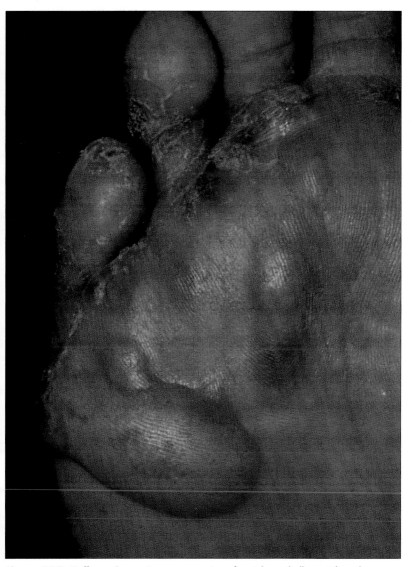

Figure 292. Bullous tinea. An acute eruption of vesicles or bullae on the sole or sides of the foot is characteristic of bullous tinea. The lesions are usually pruritic and rarely painful. Often *Trichophyton mentagrophytes* is the causative fungus. The method of bulla formation appears to be the same as that for allergic contact dermatitis.

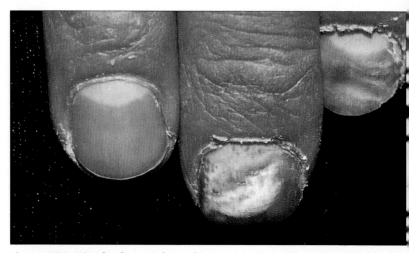

Figure 293. Distal subungual onychomycosis. Fungal organisms enter at the distal edge of the nail bed. Subungual debris accumulates, lifting the nail and causing onycholysis. Invasion of the nail plate causes it to thicken and turn yellow, brown or white. The causative agent is usually a dermatophyte but one may also find a yeast (e.g. *Candida*) or a mold (e.g. *Aspergillus*).

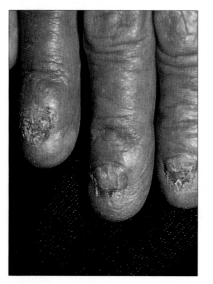

Figure 294. Chronic mucocutaneous candidiasis. In this condition, the patient suffers from chronic, recurrent infections of the nails, paronychial area, skin and mucosa by *Candida*, usually *C. albicans*. Total nail destruction commonly occurs. Various associations have included endocrinopathies, thymoma, interstitial keratitis and susceptibility to other infectious agents. Both autosomal dominant and autosomal recessive inherited forms occur.

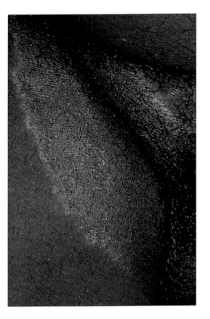

Figure 295. Tinea cruris, male. Red, scaly plaques radiating out from the inguinal fold onto the inner thigh are characteristic of tinea cruris. The border is usually scaly, raised and KOH positive. Itching may vary from absent to severe.

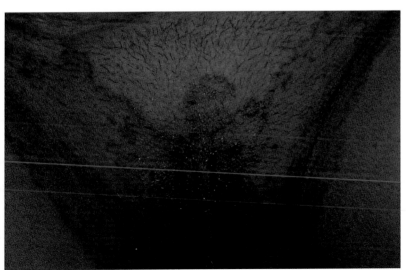

Figure 296. Tinea cruris, female. Rarely, a woman may develop a dermatophyte infection of the groin.

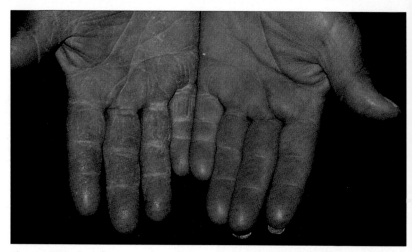

Figure 297. Two foot, one hand disease. Chronic scaling of both feet and the dominant hand secondary to a fungal infection occurs in two foot, one hand disease. Unilateral onychomycosis may be present in chronic cases. Often the patient thinks the scaling is only caused by dry skin or physical trauma. Note the diffuse scale of the right hand without inflammation.

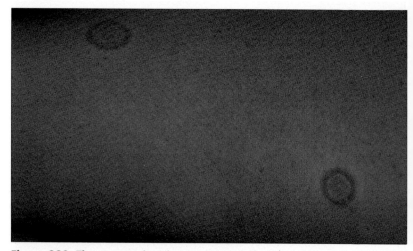

Figure 298. Tinea corporis, 'ringworm'. Multiple, large, red, scaly lesions on the body, often with an active border are characteristic. Nummular eczema, in contrast, usually shows uniform inflammation, scale and/or crust throughout. (See **Figure 227**.)

Figure 299. Tinea corporis. The entire lower part of the abdomen is affected. Note the active border and the irregular, serpiginous margin.

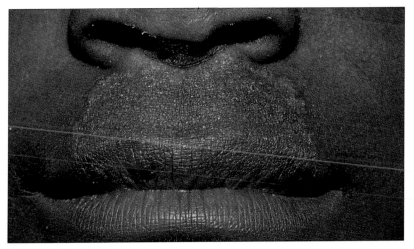

Figure 300. Tinea of the face.

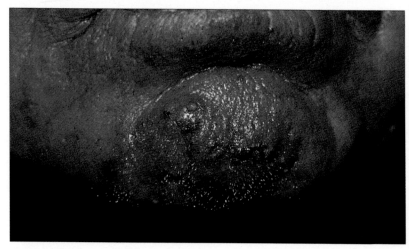

Figure 301. Tinea barbae. Fungal infection occasionally affects the beard area as annular, red, scaly rings or as aggregated follicular pustules, as shown here.

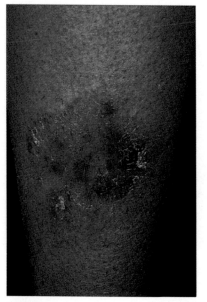

Figure 302. Majocchi's granuloma. This fungal infection (usually by *T. rubrum*) occurs deep and thus may resist topical antifungal therapy. Clinically, one sees a papulopustular perifollicular eruption on one leg of a woman who shaves. It is often mistaken for a bacterial folliculitis.

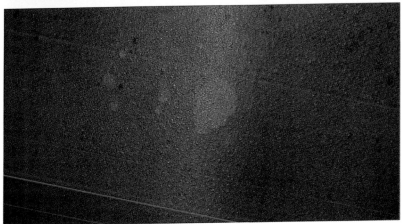

Figures 303–306 Tinea versicolor. Hyper- (**Figure 303**, top) or hypopigmented (**Figure 304**, bottom) patches on the upper back of a young adult with a slight scale when scraped (**Figure 305**, on page 162) are characteristic of tinea versicolor. The chest and neck may also be affected. Often the most bothersome aspect for the patient is the lesion's inability to tan. The most common predisposing factor is excessive sweating but others include application of oils, systemic steroids and, rarely, adrenocorticalism. A potassium hydroxide preparation of the scale (**Figure 306**, on page 162) shows short hyphae and budding cells ('spaghetti and meatballs').

See also tinea capitis (**Figures 90–93**).

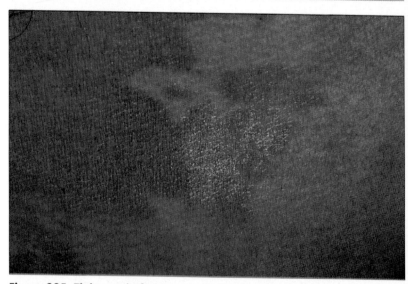

Figure 305. Tinia versicolor. Note the slight scale when scraped.

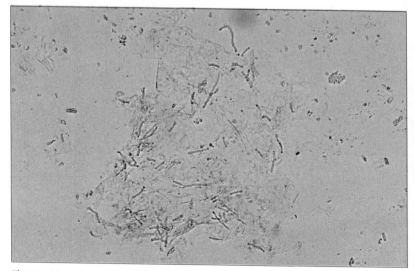

Figure 306. Tinea versicolor. 'Spaghetti and meatballs'. (Courtesy Terence C. O'Grady, MD.)

Deep Fungal and Tropical Infections

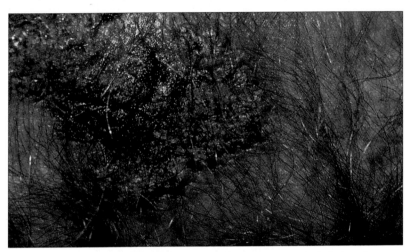

Figure 307. North American blastomycosis. Solitary or multiple lesions that begin as papulonodules and slowly enlarge to form verrucous, vegetating plaques, often with central clearing, are characteristic. Within these lesions, pustules, exudate and crust may form. Diagnosis is usually made by skin biopsy from which the organisms may be identified and cultured. The organism is *Blastomyces dermatitidis*.

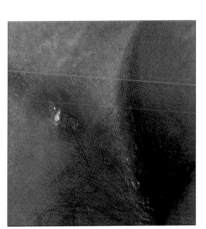

Figure 308. Coccidiomycosis.
Coccidiomycosis immitus is indigenous to the southwestern USA, Mexico and Central and South America. Cutaneous coccidiomycosis may manifest itself as multiple papulopustules, papulonodules, granulomatous papules or plaques, ulcers (as shown here) and subcutaneous abscess.

Figure 309. Cutaneous larva migrans. A red, pruritic linear eruption on the foot, back, thigh or elsewhere is characteristic of this infection by the larval nematode. In the USA, the dog or cat hookworm (*Ancylostoma caninum* or *Ancylostoma braziliense*) is a common cause. The patient acquires the infection from wet sand or dirt contaminated with animal feces.

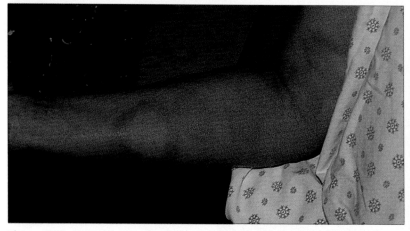

Figure 310. Leprosy, annular lesion. The classic division of leprosy is into a tuberculoid (paucibacillary, few organisms and high resistance) and a lepromatous (multibacillary, many organisms, low resistance) type with borderline between the two. The typical lesion in the tuberculoid type is a large annular erythematous plaque with an involuting, hypopigmented, anesthetic center. Nerve enlargement (e.g. greater auricular, superficial peroneal) with muscle atrophy may occur.

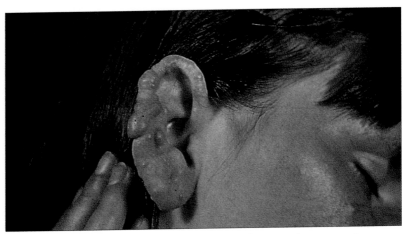

Figure 311. Leprosy, lepromatous, histiocytoid type. In lepromatous leprosy, nodular infiltration of the face, ears and elsewhere may occur. The eyebrows may be progressively lost. Note the nodular infiltration of the ear in this teenage Peruvian girl. (Courtesy of James Steger, MD.)

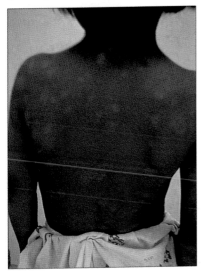

Figure 312. Leprosy, borderline tuberculoid. Note the multiple, hypopigmented lesions. (Courtesy of James Steger, MD.)

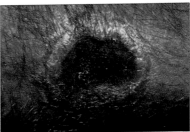

Figure 313. Leishmaniasis, ulcer. An inflammatory red–brown papulonodule develops initially at the site of a bite by the sand fly, usually on the face, neck or arms. The incubation period is usually several months but may be from a few days to over a year. The lesion enlarges to a crusted nodule. The crust may then fall off, leaving a large ulcer (as shown here on the arm) that later heals with a scar.

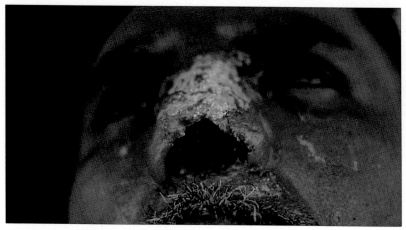

Figure 314. Leishmaniasis, nasal destruction. In a small percentage of cases, infection by *L. brasiliensis* may spread to the nasopharyngeal mucosa causing significant destruction. (Courtesy of James Steger, MD.)

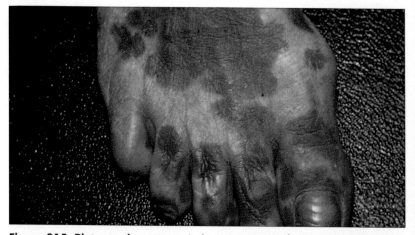

Figure 315. Pinta, tertiary stage. In the primary stage of pinta, a minute macule or papule develops at the site of inoculation and spreads to form a large 10–12.5 cm poorly defined, erythematous infiltrated plaque. In the secondary stage, pintids form that are red, violaceous, blue, brown, gray or black papulosquamous plaques. They may fade and relapse, forming polycyclic lesions. In the tertiary or late dyschromic stage of pinta, which occurs months to a decade after the pintids, depigmented patches develop as shown here. There are never systemic lesions. The organism is *Treponema carateum*. (Courtesy of James Steger, MD.)

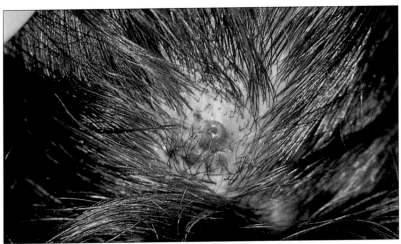

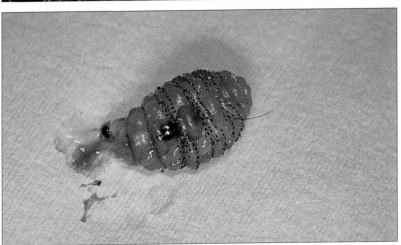

Figures 316 and 317. Myiasis. Multiple, scattered red, papulonodules much like furuncles that may drain a serosanguinous fluid (**Figure 316**, top) are characteristic of myiasis, caused by the larva of flies (**Figure 317**, bottom), order Diptera, e.g. *Dermatobia hominis*. The adult female lays eggs on the ground that hatch to first-stage larvae. They then penetrate the skin of a warm-blooded animal (e.g. a human lying on the ground or sand) and mature to adult larvae. The larvae then fall to the ground and turn into flies. (Courtesy of Stacy Smith, MD.)

Sexually Transmitted Diseases

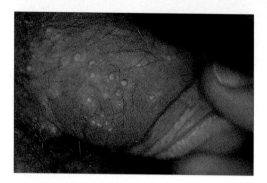

Figure 318. Molluscum contagiosum. Lesions of molluscum on the lower abdomen and groin of adults are often transmitted during sexual contact. In contrast, genital lesions in children in most cases are innocently obtained. (See also **Figure 88**.)

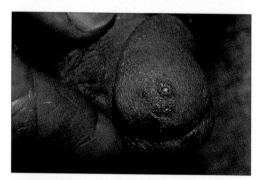

Figure 319. Herpes genitalis, male. Pain or burning may preceed by several hours the eruption of grouped vesicles on an erythematous base in herpes simplex. Primary infection is more severe than recurrences.

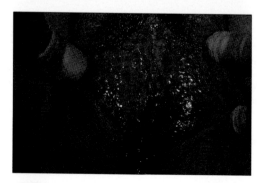

Figure 320. Herpes genitalis, female. (Courtesy of Michael O Murphy, MD.)

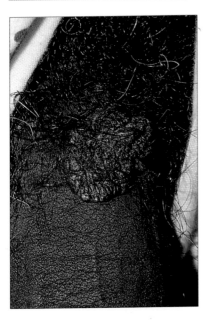

Figure 321. Condyloma acuminata, penis. Scattered, flesh-colored or hyperpigmented, smooth or verrucous papules or erythematous macules along the shaft, scrotum and perianal area are characteristic. The term bowenoid papulosis is used when the histologic picture of a lesion resembles Bowen's diseases.

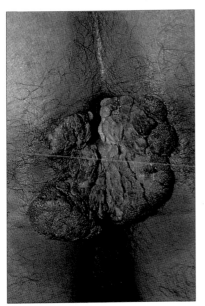

Figure 322. Condyloma acuminata, perianal. The viral particles causing perianal condyloma may have originated from warts elsewhere on the body and been transmitted via the patient's own hands, or they may have been contracted during anal sex. (See also **Figure 89**.)

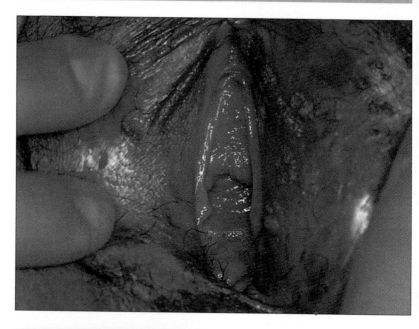

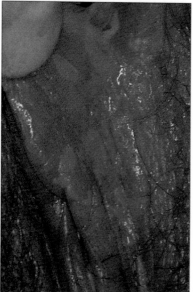

Figure 323 and 324. Vulvar intraepithelial neoplasia III. In the female genitalia, condyloma acuminata and bowenoid papulosis are sometimes grouped under the term vulvar intraepithelial neoplasia, and the atypia graded from I to III. Erythematous or pigmented, smooth or papillomatous papules, sometimes coalescent into nodules, are characteristic. Human papilloma virus, especially type 16, has been found in a significant percentage of lesions and thus the patient should be monitored for atypia of the uterine cervix. (Courtesy of Paul Koonings, MD.)

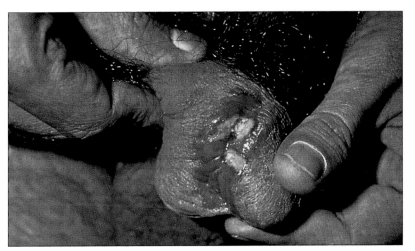

Figure 325. Primary syphilis, chancre. In primary syphilis, solitary or multiple, painless ulcers or erosions called chancres occur. They tend to remain superficial but may become indurated. In women, the chancres may occur in the vagina or on the cervix and go unnoticed. Chancres may occur at other sites of inoculation (e.g. the anus in a homosexual man, the mouth after oral sex). The organism is *Treponema pallidum*. (Courtesy of Department of Dermatology, UCSD.)

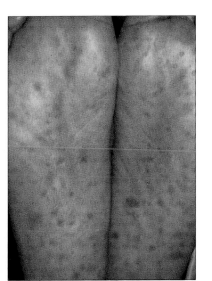

Figure 326. Secondary syphilis, papulosquamous lesions, soles. Approximately 6 weeks after the chancre, malaise, headache, fever, lymphadenopathy and a mucocutaneous eruption develop. A widespread papulosquamous eruption of ham-to-copper-hued lesions with a predilection for the palms and soles is characteristic. Scale, when present, tends to be located at the periphery. Necrotic or nodular forms occur. (Courtesy of Ted Sebastian, MD.)

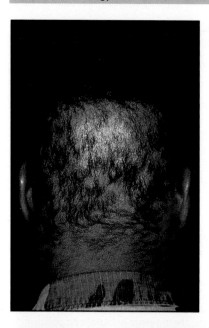

Figure 327. Secondary syphilis, moth-eaten alopecia. Patchy, 'moth-eaten' alopecia affects the scalp, eyebrows, eyelashes and beard. (Courtesy of Stacy Smith, MD.)

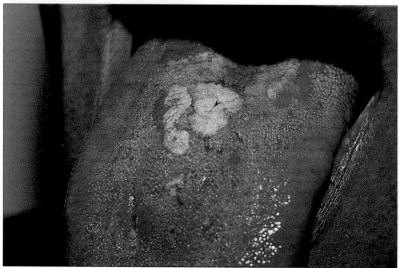

Figure 328. Secondary syphilis, mucous patch. Whitish-grey papules and plaques may occur on the tongue, or other mucous membrane surfaces.

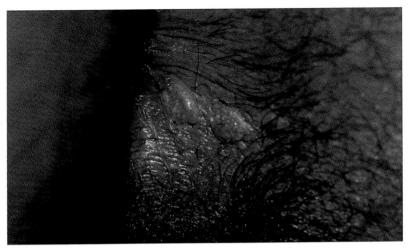

Figure 329. Secondary syphilis, condyloma lata, perianal. These lesions are teeming with *T. pallidum.*

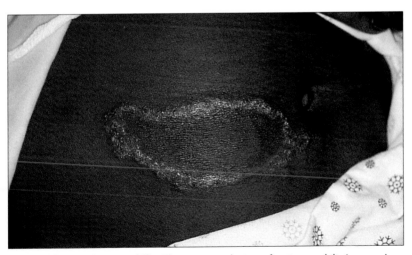

Figure 330. Tertiary syphilis. The cutaneous lesions of tertiary syphilis (gummas) are often polycyclic or serpiginous with central ulceration or clearing. These granulomatous lesions are usually painless but may be locally destructive. Gummatous lesions may develop internally as well. (Courtesy of Department of Dermatology, UCSD.)

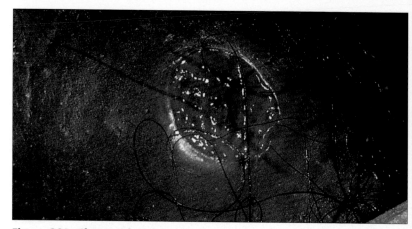

Figure 331. Chancroid. *Haemophilus ducreyi* causes chancroid. On smear it has a 'school of fish' appearance, and lesions tend to be painful and foul smelling. Several other infectious organisms may cause a genital ulcer. *Calymmatobacterium granulomatosis* causes granuloma inguinale, also known as donovanosis. The ulcer tends to be beefy yet asymptomatic with exuberant granulation tissue. *Chlamydia trachomatis* causes lymphogranuloma venerium. The genital lesion typically is a small erosion that goes unnoticed. One to two weeks later, firm lymphadenopathy develops. The classic 'groove' sign is created by enlarged inguinal and femoral nodes separated by Poupart's ligament. (Courtesy of Stacy Smith, MD.)

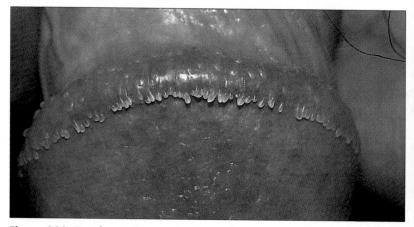

Figure 332. Pearly penile papules. Two or three rows of uniform, flesh-colored papules running circumferentially about the corona are characteristic. Onset is typically noted in the 20s and 30s. These papules may be mistaken for warts but are not infectious.

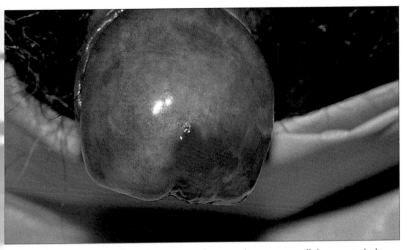

Figure 333. Zoon's balanitis. A moist, shiny, erythematous, well-demarcated plaque on the glans penis in an older uncircumcised male is characteristic of Zoon's balanitis, also known as balanitis plasmocellularis. The condition is benign.

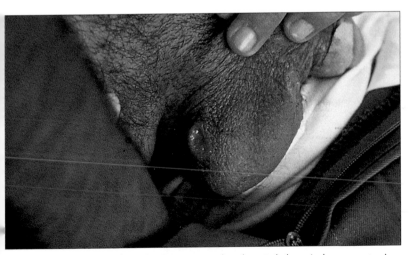

Figure 334. Behçet's disease. Recurrent oral and genital ulcers (vulva or scrotum) occur in Behçet's disease. Other organ systems that are affected include the eye (e.g. relapsing iridocyclitis), CNS (e.g. meningoencephalitis), joints and skin (e.g. erythema nodosum-like, vasculitic or papulopustular lesions). (Courtesy of Erkan Alpsoy, MD.)

Viral Infections

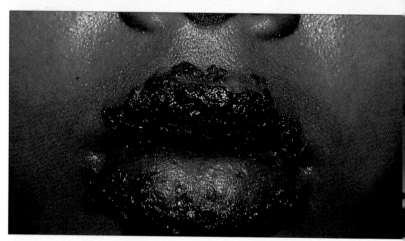

Figure 335. Herpes labialis, primary. This crusting, vesicular primary herpes simplex virus (HSV) infection of the lips and/or the oropharynx is most common in children. Fever and lymphodenopathy may occur. HSV-1 is the predominant pathogen.

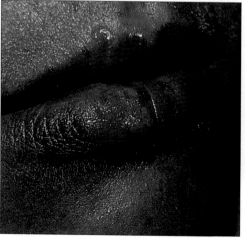

Figure 336. Herpes labialis, recurrent. Pain or tingling followed by grouped vesicles on an erythematous base on the lip, typically centered on the vermilion border but also on nearby sites, is characteristic of this recurrent infection by HSV. Triggering factors for herpes labialis include dental work, fever, UV radiation, local trauma, mental stress or menstruation.

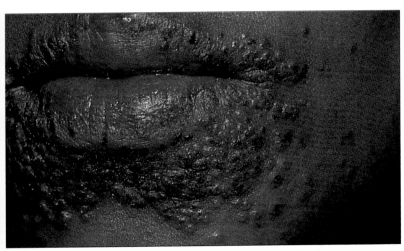

Figure 337 Eczema herpeticum. Atopic skin seems particularly susceptible to infection by herpes simplex. It is signaled by the acute eruption of diffuse vesicles that quickly rupture leaving erosions and crusting. (See also **Figures 50 and 51**.)

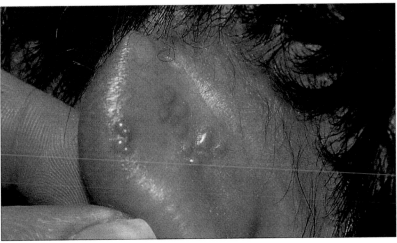

Figure 338. Herpes simplex, pustular. After several days, the clear vesicles of herpes become pustules.

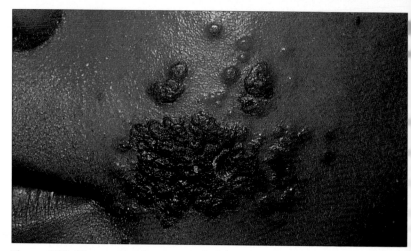

Figure 339. Herpes simplex, crusted. The crusting of herpes is often mistaken for impetigo, especially in children. Always look for intact vesicles and pustules among the crust. Bacterial and viral cultures are invaluable.

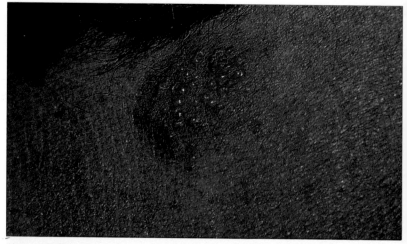

Figure 340. Herpes zoster, early mimicking herpes simplex. This patient presented with this isolated group of painful vesicles on an erythematous base. Herpes simplex was suspected. It was only when the patient returned 2 days later (**Figure 341**) with multiple lesions scattered in a dermatome that the correct diagnosis of herpes zoster was made.

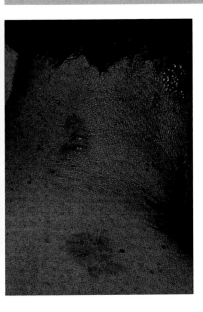

Figure 341. Herpes zoster. Groups of vesicles, each on an erythematous base scattered within a dermatome, are characteristic. The trunk and face are most commonly affected. The lesions stop at the midline. Intense pain may incapacitate the patient. A few lesions may be found outside the dermatome, however, generalization of the zoster may occur, especially in those with decreased cellular immunity. Post-herpetic neuralgia (defined as pain beyond 4 weeks) is a potentially debilitating sequelae. The risk of it developing goes up significantly after the age of 60.

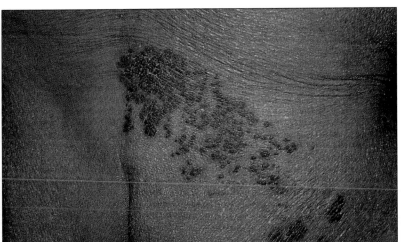

Figure 342. Herpes zoster, hemorrhagic. The vesicles of herpes zoster may at times be hemorrhagic.

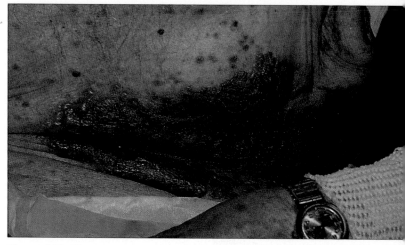

Figure 343. Herpes zoster, necrotic. In debilitated patients, necrosis may occasionally occur.

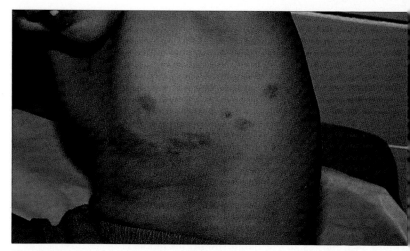

Figure 344. Herpes zoster in a child. Herpes zoster occurred in this 3-year-old girl. She had chicken pox at eighteen months. The varicella zoster virus causes both conditions. Spontaneous resolution can be expected.

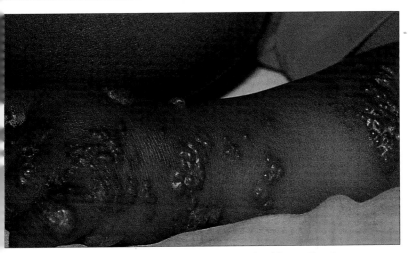

Figure 345. Herpes zoster in immunocompromised host. Shingles preferentially affects those with decreased cellular immunity, e.g. elderly people, HIV-positive patients and those with hematologic malignancy. This 3-year-old with leukemia developed shingles on the left arm.

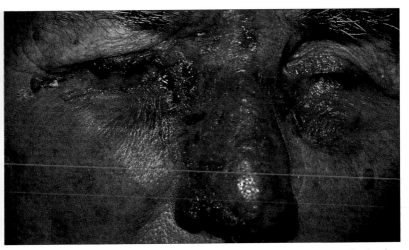

Figure 346. Ophthalmologic zoster. Vesicles and crusting of the top and side of the nose in herpes zoster implies involvement of the nasociliary branch of the trigeminal nerve and eye involvement. Ocular scarring and loss of vision may occur.

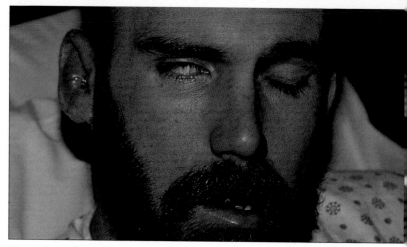

Figure 347. Ramsay–Hunt syndrome. Herpes zoster of the geniculate ganglion resulting in vesicles of the ear (shown here) and tympanic membrane occurs in Ramsay–Hunt syndrome. Both the 7th and 8th cranial nerve functions may be affected. Patients may have tinnitus, deafness, nausea, vomiting, nystagmus, facial hemiplegia and partial loss of taste. The patient shown is trying to close both eyes.

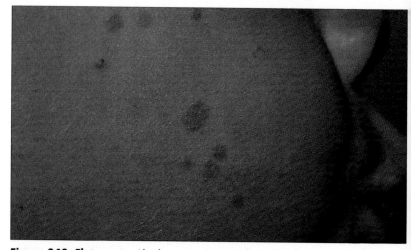

Figure 348. Flat warts. Also known as verruca plana, flat warts present as pink, flesh-colored or tan, flat-topped, slightly elevated papules common on the forehead, face and dorsa of the hands and legs. The lesions are typically caused by HPV 3. These lesions on the right cheek of a child were mistaken for multiple nevi.

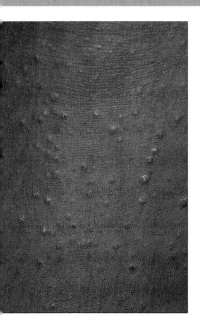

Figure 349. Flat warts, legs. The shaved legs of teenage women are commonly affected by flat warts. The razor seems to spread the infection. Tiny papules around many of the hairs are seen.

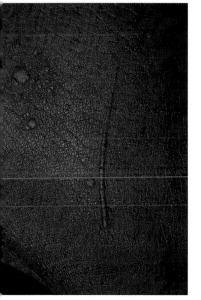

Figure 350. Flat warts, Koebnerization. Koebnerization refers to the development of a disease at the site of epidermal injury. Here scratching has caused the warts to form in a line.

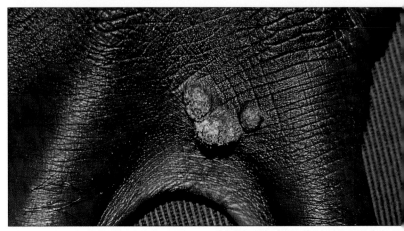

Figure 351. Verruca vulgaris. Solitary or multiple hyperkeratotic or verrucous papules on the hands or fingers of a child or adolescent are characteristic. The normal skin lines are obscured. Warts on the hands are very common and may affect all ages but with the preponderance from age 5–25 years. Even though the patient pictured is Black, verrucae seem to be more common in Whites.

Figure 352. Plantar wart. A hyperkeratotic, verrucous papule or plaque beneath a pressure point on the sole of the foot is characteristic. Paring reveals black dots, which represent thrombosed capillaries. HPV types 1 (myrmecia), 2 (mosaic) and 4 are most common. Because plantar warts are driven into the skin by the pressure of walking or standing, they are usually the most resistant to treatment.

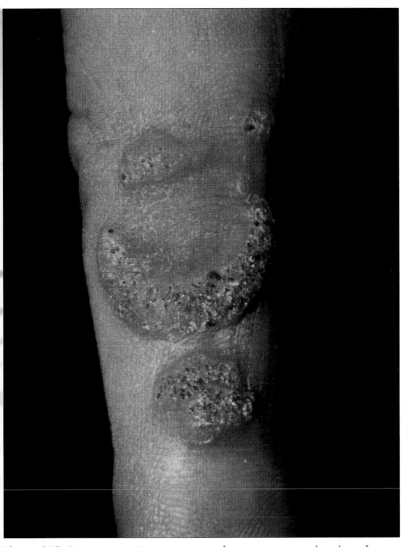

Figure 353. Donut wart. It is not uncommon for warts to recur at the edges of cryotherapy, creating the shape of a donut. (The middle lesion pictured here perhaps resembles more a crescent roll.)

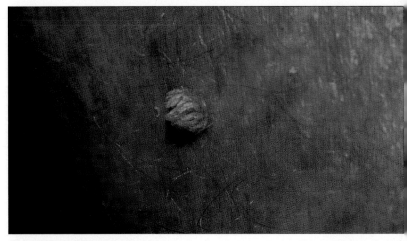

Figure 354. Filiform wart. Filiform warts are common on the face and neck of adults. Their shape is reminiscent of a horse's tail.

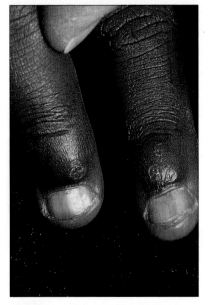

Figure 355. Verruca, periungual. Warts about the nails are common in children. Their presence may depress the matrix, causing a groove in the nail. Care must be taken to not damage the matrix when treating such verrucae, or else permanent damage to the nail may result.

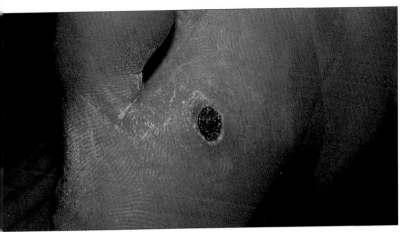

Figure 356. Regressing plantar wart. Spontaneous blackening of a plantar wart is a sign of imminent regression. It is as if the immune system suddenly did not like the wart and decided to get rid of it. Erythema and pruritis may preceed this color change. After turning black, the wart just peels and falls off.

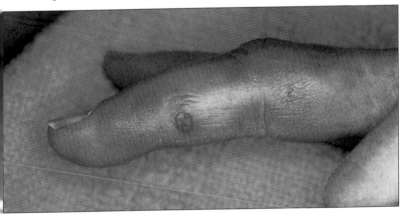

Figure 357. Orf. A solitary papulonodule develops at the site of inoculation of this zoonosis acquired from sheep or goats, also known as ecthyma contagiosa. Fever, lymphadenopathy and erythema multiforme may accompany the lesion. The causative agent is a virus from the pox virus group. (Courtesy of Eliot Mostow, MD.)

See also neonatal herpes (**Figure 31**), molluscum contagiosum (**Figure 88**), measles (**Figure 107**), roseola (**Figure 110**), chickenpox (**Figure 123**), and hand, foot and mouth disease (**Figure 125**).

Infestations and Bites

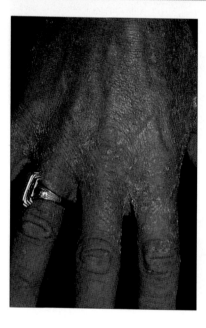

Figure 358. Scabies, hand. All patients whose predominant complaint is itching should have their web spaces, wrists and feet examined. Occasionally, the patient with scabies will complain only of a hand dermatitis or a penile eruption. The patient should fully disrobe to allow also examination of the axilla, trunk, waist, and groin. Linear, thread-like burrows often with a black dot at one end (the mite) are virtually diagnostic. A mineral examination is confirmatory. Over time, lichenification, excoriations, scabetic nodules and secondary bacterial infection may develop. The pruritus is caused by allergy to the mite, its eggs and feces. This diagnosis may be very difficult to make in the patient who scratches away the burrows. Close-up examination of the scaly lesions in this patient shows many of them to be linear.

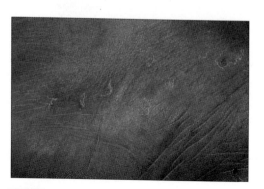

Figure 359. Scabies, burrow. The sides of the feet are excellent places to find burrows. Note the linear, thread-like, serpiginous scale.

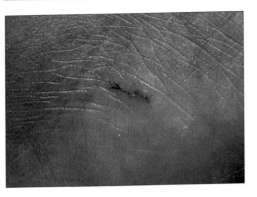

Figure 360. Scabies, burrow, ink test. The ink test is performed by rubbing the skin with black ink and then wiping it off. If burrows are present, the ink will run down into them and remain. Note the V-shaped ending of this burrow at 10 o'clock. This is where the skin is shedding the last remnants of that portion of the burrow. The end pointing to 4 o'clock is where the scabies mite is still actively burrowing.

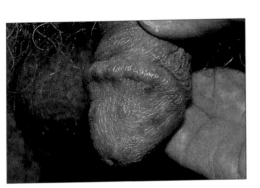

Figure 361. Scabies, nodular lesions, penis. The penis is almost always affected in some fashion by scabies in men. Nodular lesions, as shown here, often develop.

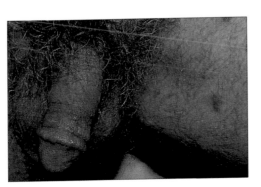

Figure 362. Scabies, nodular lesions, thigh. Multiple red–brown papulonodules may develop in the patient who has had scabies for several months. Both the penis and inner thigh are affected in this patient.

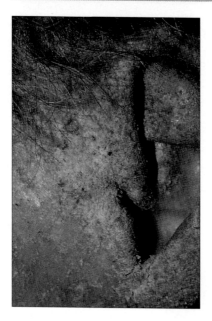

Figure 363. Crusted scabies.
Scaling, crusting and itching beginning on the hands, feet, and groin and progressing to cover the entire body are characteristic. Thousands of mites have populated the skin in contrast to conventional scabies in which the number is thought to be less than 20. Patients usually have neurologic disease (e.g. Down's syndrome, mental retardation) or immunosuppression (e.g. AIDS, hematologic malignancy).

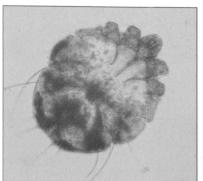

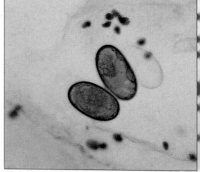

Figure 364. Scabies, microscopic examination. Affected skin is scraped with a blade moistened with mineral oil. The resultant mix is applied to a slide, covered with a cover-slip and examined microscopically. The presence of even a single mite (left), egg or scybala (right) is diagnostic.

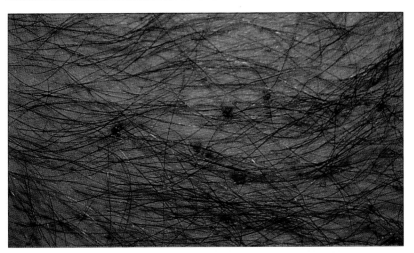

Figure 365. Pediculosis pubis, abdomen. Pruritus of the groin is often the only symptom of pediculosis pubis. Inspection of the area shows small, ovoid nits (eggs) attached firmly to the hair and pointing away from the skin. Closer inspection will show crab-like organisms hanging to the base of adjacent hairs. The organisms may spread upward to the abdomen and chest as shown here. This disease is spread by close physical (e.g. sexual) contact.

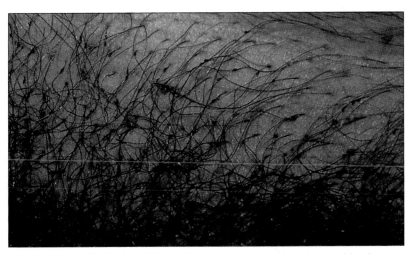

Figure 366. Pediculosis pubis, groin. Pubic, head and body lice are blood-sucking and host-specific for humans. The technical name for pubic lice is *Phthirus pubis*.

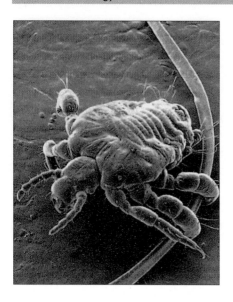

Figure 367. Pediculosis pubis. The pubic louse is shown here. (Courtesy of Morse, Moreland and Holmes (1996) *Atlas of Sexually Transmitted Diseases and AIDS*, Mosby-Wolfe.)

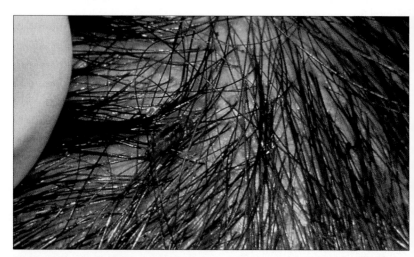

Figure 368. Pediculosis capitis, adult. Lice suck the patient's blood and leave behind digestive material and feces. Intense pruritus results. Secondary infection and alopecia from scratching may occur. Head and body lice are caused by distinct variants of *Pediculosis humanis*.

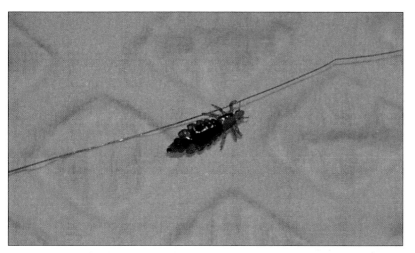

Figure 369. Pediculosis capitis, louse. Close inspection of the hair reveals the wingless louse. Note that the head and body louse have longer, slender bodies than the pubic louse which is more crab-like.

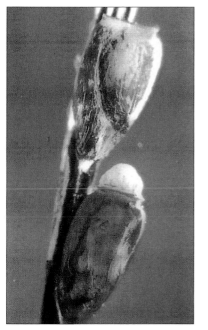

Figure 370. Pediculosis capitis, nit. The egg (nit) is shown firmly cemented to the hair shaft. (Courtesy of Morse, Moreland and Holmes (1996) *Atlas of Sexually Transmitted Diseases and AIDS*, Mosby-Wolfe.)

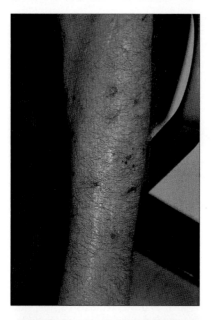

Figure 371. Pediculosis corporis.
Excoriations, crusting and urticarial papules may be seen in pediculosis corporis. The lice live on the clothes and descend on to the skin to feed. Any part of the skin covered by clothes may be affected. Usually it is the homeless or other indigent patients who do not routinely wash their clothes that are affected.

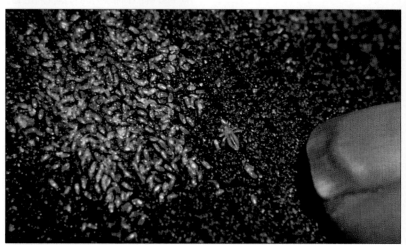

Figure 372. Pediculosis corporis, clothing plus louse. Inspection of the clothing allows for diagnosis.

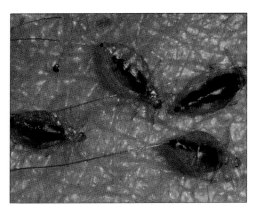

Figure 373. Pediculosis corporis, louse. (Courtesy of Peters and Gilles (1995) *Color Atlas of Tropical Medicine and Parasitology,* 4e, Mosby-Wolfe.)

Analysis of the specimens sent to us on February 26, 1993 revealed the following:

    Dry scalp   _____

    Lice   _____

    Mites   _____

    Ants   _____

    Slugs   _____

    Other   _____

Your diligence in obtaining and mailing these "bugs" for our examination is appreciated.

Sincerely,

Mr. White
Dermatology Department

Figure 374. Delusions of parasitosis. The patient is convinced that some sort of parasite or 'bug' is living in or on his or her skin. It may arise as a primary condition or secondary to a variety of disorders including drug use (e.g. alcohol, cocaine or amphetamines), organic brain dysfunction or schizophrenia. The physician must always rule out true infestation, e.g. by scabies, pediculosis, the rat mite, bird mite, etc. This author once saw an elderly woman who complained of ants crawling on her skin. When asked to bring them in, she did! Fumigating the house cured the problem. Patients may be encouraged to bring in specimens for microscopic examination. This patient even provided a form to fill out!

Figure 375. Arthropod bite. Spiders, mosquitoes or other arthropods may bite almost any part of the body. The individual papules are red, grouped and intensely itchy. The bug whose bites are shown here had breakfast, lunch, dinner and a snack!

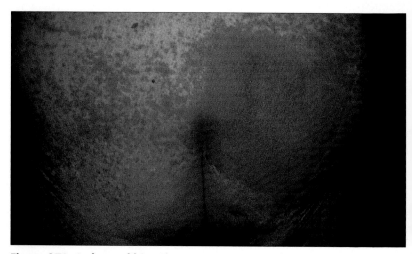

Figure 376. Arthropod bite. The immune response to a bite may be dramatic as shown in this woman who was bitten on the right buttock.

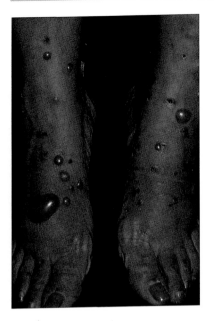

Figure 377. Flea bite, bulla. Flea bites occur about the ankles because these tiny brown insects can jump no higher than 2 feet (60 cm). Vesicles and bullae may occur. Because the host's immune response is important in pathogenesis, only one member of the family may be affected. (See also **Figure 97**.)

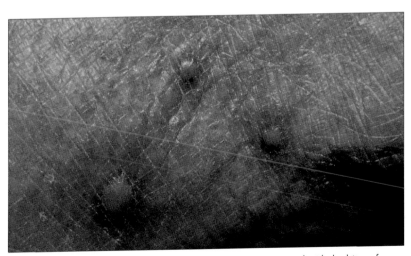

Figure 378. Fire ants. Intense burning and pain are associated with the bites of these ants. A wheal is followed by a vesicle, which finally forms a pustule as shown here. This woman had stepped on a group of ants 7 days before presenting.

Inflammatory Disorders

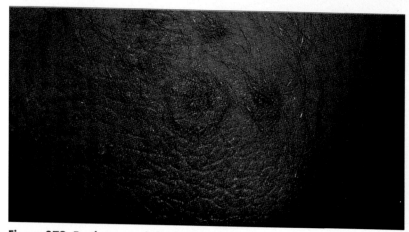

Figure 379. Erythema multiforme, target lesion. Multiple target lesions (concentric rings of different shades of red) often with a dusky, necrotic or bullous center occur in erythema multiforme. The dorsum of the hand is one of the most commonly affected sites. Implicated causes are legion but a recent herpes infection is most common.

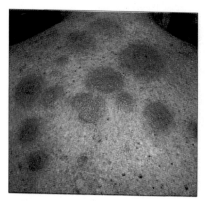

Figure 380. Sweet's syndrome. Also known as acute febrile neutrophilic dermatosis, Sweet's syndrome may present with fever, leukocytosis and rapidly developing painful, red plaques on the upper back, arms, face, neck or elsewhere. The abdomen, lower back, buttocks and posterior thighs tend to be spared. The surface of these plaques may exhibit a mamillated appearance, pustules, pseudovesiculation or crusting. Erythema nodosum-like lesions may occur on the legs and arms. (Courtesy of Michael O Murphy, MD.)

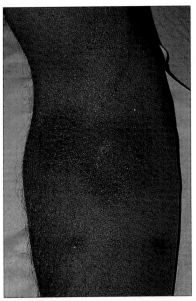

Figure 381. Well's syndrome. Acute attacks of erythematous plaques—resembling cellulitis—are characteristic. Multiple recurrences are common, and this condition may be misdiagnosed as recurrent cellulitis for years. Blood eosinophilia is a frequent but not required sign.

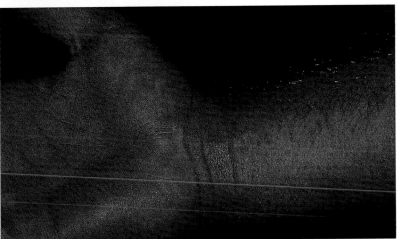

Figure 382. Gloves and socks syndrome. Confluent erythema of the palms and soles that stops at the wrists and ankles is characteristic. Significant purpura often occurs. Lymphadenopathy, leukopenia, fever and oral erythema or erosion may occur. This rash seems to be a viral exanthem, associated most commonly with parvovirus B19, but also to other viruses.

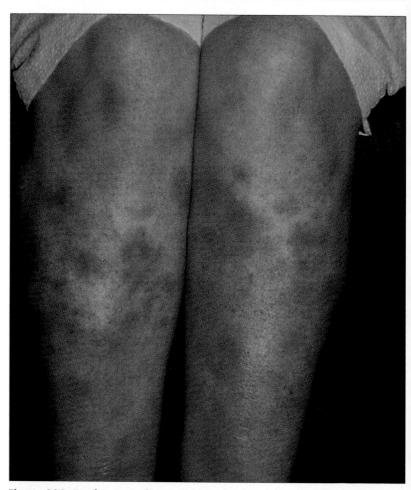

Figure 383. Erythema nodosum. Red, tender, deep-seated nodules scattered on both shins in an adult are characteristic. The disease usually runs its course over 3–6 weeks. Precipitating factors include various infections (e.g. streptococcal, tuberculosis, coccidiomycosis (shown here), blastomycosis, histoplasmosis, *Yersinia*, salmonella enteritis, Chlamydia, milker's nodules, tularemia and hepatitis B), drugs (e.g. birth control pills), pregnancy, ulcerative colitis, sarcoidosis and rarely malignancy, e.g. lymphoma. Both Sweet's syndrome and cryoglobulinemia can cause lesions that resemble erythema nodosum. Work-up may include skin biopsy, complete blood count, urine analysis, antistreptolysin-O, throat culture, chest X-ray, liver enzymes, stool culture if diarrhea is present and intradermal or serologic tests for deep fungi.

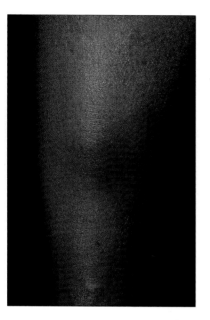

Figure 384. Villanova's disease. A painless, erythematous nodule enlarging to a plaque on the lower aspect of one shin in a woman is characteristic of Villanova's disease, also called subacute nodular migratory panniculitis. The lesion may be chronic with slow expansion. The lesion is usually misdiagnosed as cellulitis. Many consider this disease a variant of erythema nodosum and use the term erythema nodosum migrans.

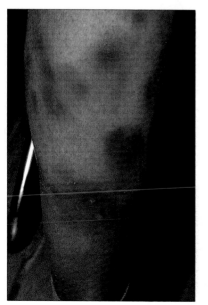

Figure 385. Nodular vasculitis. Tender, red, deep-seated nodules, mainly on the calves, chiefly in women are characteristic. Ulceration commonly occurs. A work-up to exclude tuberculosis should be done. If tuberculosis is found, the term erythema induratum of Bazin is used.

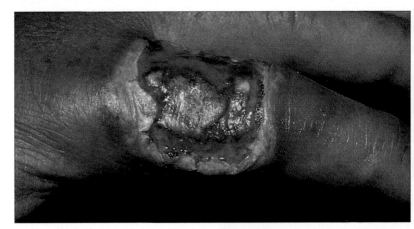

Figure 386. Pyoderma gangrenosum, ulcer, dorsa hand. Pyoderma gangrenosum is a non-infectious ulcerative disease classically associated with chronic inflammatory conditions such as ulcerative colitis, Crohn's disease, arthritis, chronic active hepatitis and Takayasu's arteritis. In making the diagnosis, infection (e.g. deep fungal), malignancy (e.g. lymphoma) and vasculopathy (e.g. Wegener's granulomatosis, antiphospholipid syndrome) must be excluded.

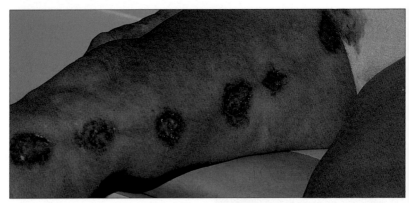

Figure 387. Pyoderma gangrenosum, multiple ulcers. Beginning as a papule or pustule, the lesion breaks down to form an ulcer with an undermined, violaceous, jagged border. It commonly occurs on the legs but also elsewhere—and is often painful. Lesions may occur at sites of trauma (pathergy) as shown here after surgery. Work-up may include antinuclear antibodies (ANA), rheumatoid factor, hepatic and renal enzymes, complete blood count, rapid plasma reagin, serum protein electrophoresis, evaluation of the gastrointestinal tract and biopsy of the margin of the ulcer for histopathology and culture (e.g. bacterial, viral, fungal, atypical mycobacteria).

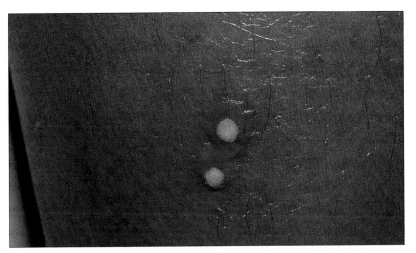

Figure 388. Pyoderma gangrenosum, pustule. The earliest sign of pyoderma gangrenosum may be a pustule.

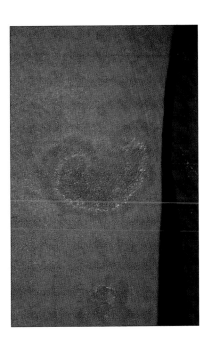

Figure 389. Erythema annulare centrificum. Annular red lesions with a classic trailing scale are characteristic of erythema annulare centrificum. The morphology is distinct from tinea corporis, which classically has a scaly leading edge. Two clinical subtypes are recognized, a superficial gyrate erythema (scaly, pruritic) and a deep gyrate erythema (non-pruritic, non-scaly, annular, red) (see **Figures 390–392**). Work-up includes a search for any antigenic stimulus, such as tinea pedis, a new drug, blue-cheese ingestion (contains penicillin). streptococcal infection, thyroid disease, dental infection, viral infection (e.g. Epstein–Barr virus) or malignancy.

Figure 390. Gyrate erythema. This and the following two photographs were taken at approximately 3 week intervals and illustrate the deep variant of erythema annulare centrificum. The initial lesion is an erythematous, urticarial papule or plaque.

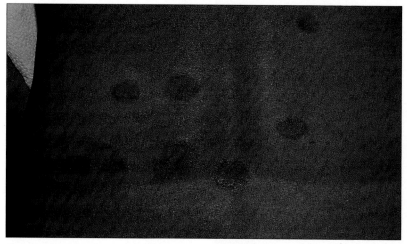

Figure 391. Gyrate erythema.

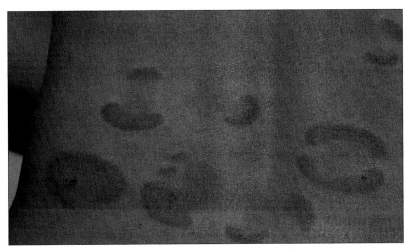

Figure 392. Gyrate erythema. By the sixth week, annular lesions have formed. Most lesions have had part of their circle resolve leaving various arcs and post-inflammatory hyperpigmentation.

Figure 393. Jessner's lymphocytic infiltrate. Erythematous, red, non-scaly, infiltrated papules, plaques and arcs on the face, arms and trunk occur in Jessner's lymphocytic infiltrate. It is most common in adults, but may rarely affect children. ANA and Ro (ss-A) autoantibody should be checked, and a biopsy performed.

Figure 394. Granuloma annulare. Initially, a red dermal papule forms and spreads outward, involuting centrally. Later, multiple dermal papules linked together form spreading, annular rings. Granuloma annulare is most common on the dorsa of the hands but lesions occur elsewhere (e.g. the elbows, fingers, palms, dorsa of the feet, etc.).

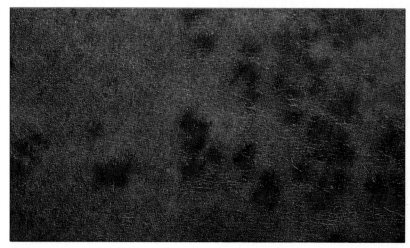

Figure 395. Granuloma annulare. A disseminated form, consisting of hundreds of papules and/or annular lesions spread across the trunk, may occur. It may be associated with diabetes.

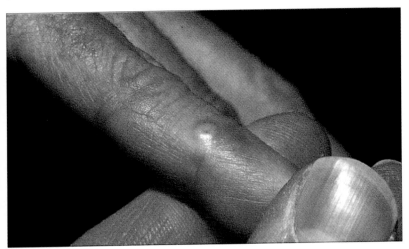

Figure 396. Granuloma annulare. Some variants of granuloma annulare are characterized by papules with a central dell.

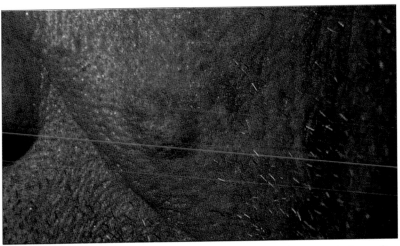

Figure 397. Granuloma faciale. A red–brown plaque or plaques on the face, often with a peau d'orange surface is characteristic. The nose is often involved and middle-aged white men are most often affected.

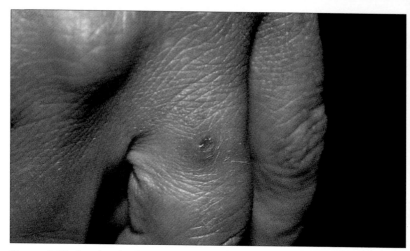

Figure 398. Foreign body, papule. Foreign bodies may produce inflammatory reactions in the skin. This patient presented with the solitary violaceous papule as shown. She denied a history of trauma.

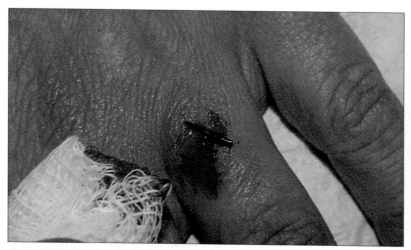

Figure 399. Foreign body, biopsy of showing thorn. Only after biopsy and extraction of a thorn did the patient remember being 'stuck' by a Yucca plant 4.5 years before. To make the story even more surprising, the initial injury occurred 4–5 cm away on the dorsa of the hand.

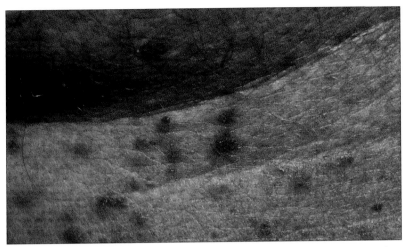

Figure 400. Grover's disease. Discrete, truncal pruritic papules and papulovesicles in a middle-aged or elderly person are characteristic of Grover's disease, also known as transient acantholytic dermatosis. Although usually transient (weeks to months), the disease may also last years.

Figure 401. Itchy red bump disease. An adult with chronic pruritus and 1–2 mm erythematous papulovesicles scattered on the body is characteristic. The diagnosis of this disease is one of exclusion. Scabies preparation, patch testing, drug history, skin biopsy and a trial of antibiotics are helpful to exclude scabies, Grover's disease, allergic contact dermatitis, drug rash, dermatitis herpetiformis and folliculitis.

Keratoses, Tags and Fibromas

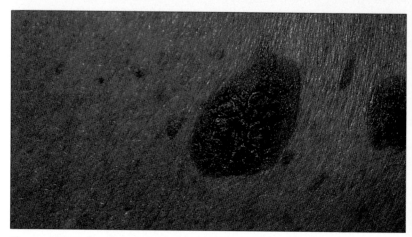

Figure 402. Seborrheic keratosis. These brown, stuck-on, warty, papules or plaques are found on almost every older adult and have been called 'barnacles on the ship of life'. They may be dark brown or black, light tan or white, nearly flat or raised, smooth and greasy or rough and warty. Almost any area of the body may be affected.

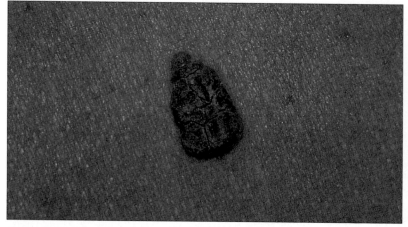

Figure 403. Seborrheic keratosis.

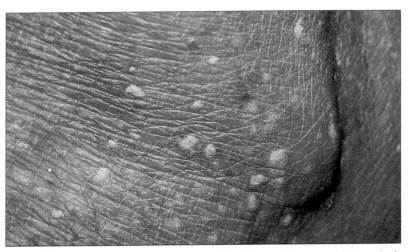

Figure 404. Stucco keratosis. This variant of a seborrheic keratosis is distinguished by its white color and preference for the tops of the feet and/or ankles in an older adult.

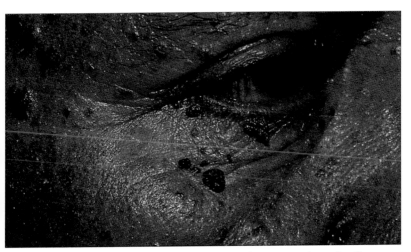

Figure 405. Dermatosis papulosa nigra. Multiple, pigmented papules, flat or filiform on the face and neck of a darker-skinned person are characteristic.

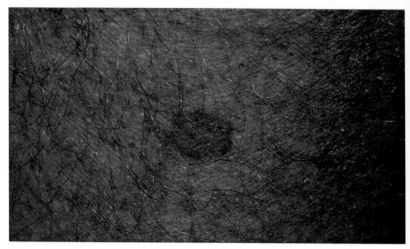

Figure 406. Benign lichenoid keratosis. The classic story is that of a brown spot, present for months to years that suddenly becomes red, inflamed, slightly raised and itchy. It is as if the body suddenly decides to go on the attack.

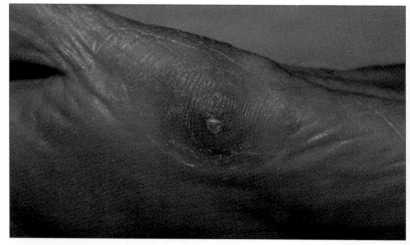

Figure 407. Corn. This hyperkeratotic, painful papule on the sole, dorsa of the toes or in the web spaces is the result of repeated pressure. An underlying bony prominence or exostosis is always found. Direct pressure causes pain.

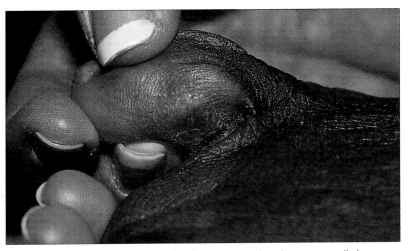

Figure 408. Soft corn. Soft corns develop in the interdigital spaces, usually between the 4th and 5th toes, and are so called because the hyperkeratotic skin is hydrated and soft.

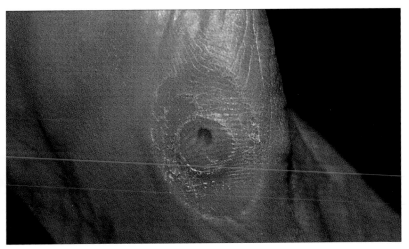

Figure 409. Corn, pared. Paring of a corn reveals the characteristic translucent core - in contrast to a wart which shows black dots and bleeding (**Figure 410**).

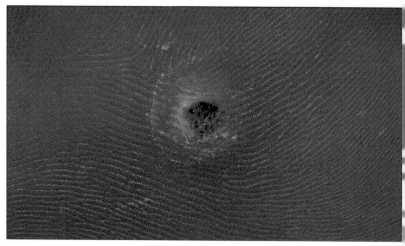

Figure 410. Verruca. In contrast to a corn (**Figure 409**) , paring a verruca reveals black dots and bleeding. The black dots represent thrombosed capillaries. (See also **Figures 351–356**.)

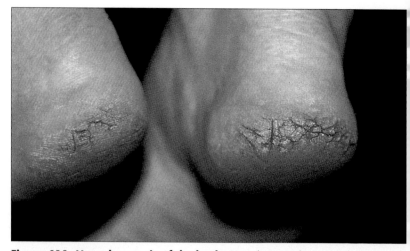

Figure 411. Hyperkeratosis of the heels. Hyperkeratosis beginning laterally, with potential progression to cover the entire heel, is common in middle-aged patients. Some have ascribed causes of faulty walking technique, pressure, sandals and ill-fitting shoes.

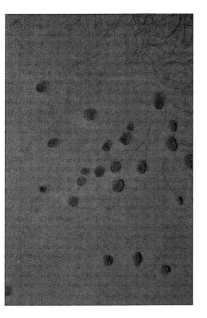

Figure 412. Skin tags. Pedunculated or filiform, fleshy, pink or brown papules 1–10 mm on the sides of the neck, axilla, eyelids or groin in a middle-aged or older adult are characteristic of skin tags, also called acrochordons. Patients often complain that tags on the neck catch on collars or necklaces. The presence of skin tags positively correlates with weight, height and colonic polyps.

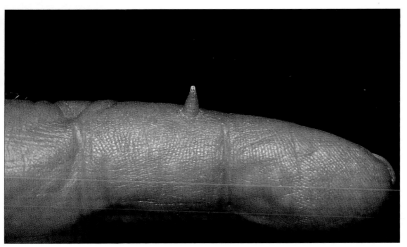

Figure 413. Acquired digital fibrokeratoma. These flesh-colored papules on the finger, usually index or middle finger, are characteristically mistaken for warts. One telltale feature that distinguishes it from a wart is an epidermal collarette at its base. These lesions may also occur on the toes, palms or heels.

Nail Disorders

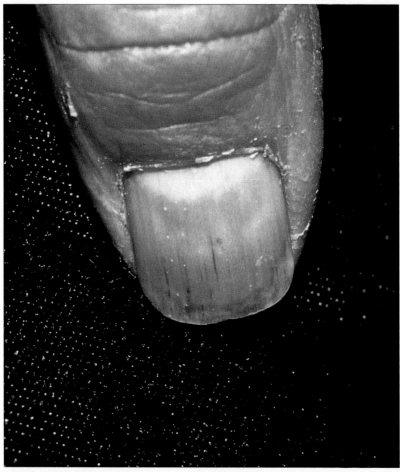

Figure 414. Splinter hemorrhage. A longitudinal linear, red or black streak below the nail is characteristic. Common 'benign' splinter hemorrhages occur in the middle or distal nail bed and are black. They are common in elderly people. This contrasts with the rarer splinter hemorrhages associated with systemic disease (e.g. subacute bacterial endocarditis) that occur more proximally and are red.

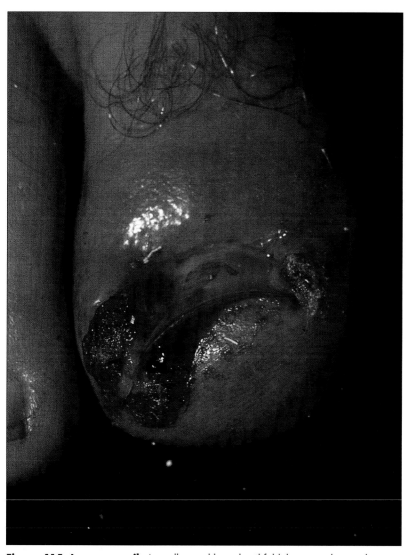

Figure 415. Ingrown nail. A swollen, red lateral nail fold that extends over the lateral edge of the nail is characteristic. The nail burrows into the lesion causing a foreign body response, producing more swelling. The big toe is most commonly affected. Secondary bacterial infection occurs.

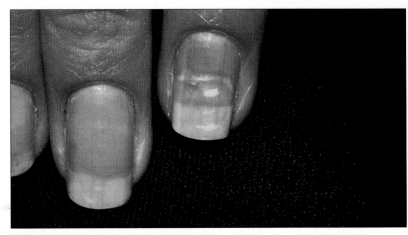

Figure 416. Onycholysis. Separation of the nail plate from the bed is called onycholysis and is most commonly seen in women. Causes include psoriasis (look for pits, family history, oil spots), trauma (ask if they are cleaning under nails and with what?) photo-onycholysis (e.g. from tetracycline or less commonly psoralens), allergic contact dermatitis (from nail products such as hardeners or polish), systemic causes (e.g. thyroid abnormalities, pregnancy) and fungal infection (e.g. *Candida*). Women with onycholysis of long fingernails and no other obvious cause may have developed them secondary to chronic lifting of the nail off the bed during the course of normal activity.

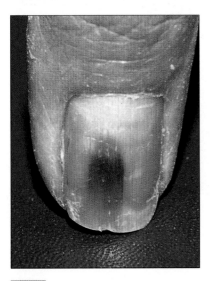

Figure 417. *Pseudomonas.* A green discoloration of the nail occurs when the space created by onycholysis is colonized by *Pseudomonas*.

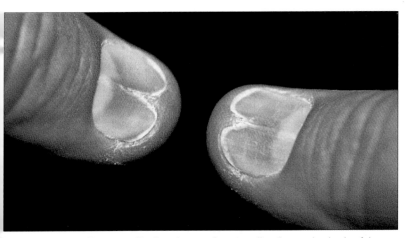

Figure 418. Median canalicular dystrophy. A midline longitudinal split of the nail (usually the thumb nail) occurs in median canalicular dystrophy. Lines extending outward on both sides give the appearance of a fur tree.

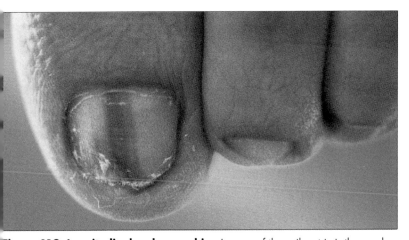

Figure 419. Longitudinal melanonychia. A nevus of the nail matrix is the usual cause of this pigmented streak of the nail but an atypical nevus or a melanoma must be excluded. A wide, dark, solitary band in an older person should be biopsied, whereas multiple narrow bands uniformly colored in a dark-skinned young person are likely to be benign (See **Figure 170**). Pigmentation of the periungual skin (Hutchison's sign) is particularly worrisome. (Courtesy of Steven Goldberg, MD.)

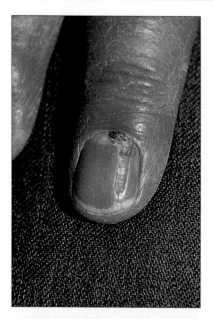

Figure 420. Digital mucous cyst, groove. A longitudinal groove of the nail plate may develop from any growth or tumor which pushes down on the nail matrix. The digital mucous cyst is most common but a glomus tumor may be found as well.

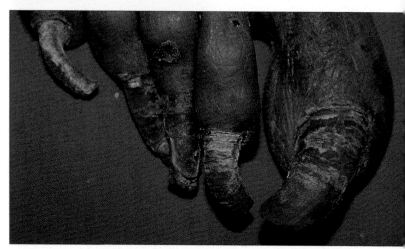

Figure 421. Onychogryphosis. Opaque, thickened nails with exaggerated growth upward and/or laterally are characteristic of nail hypertrophy. Old age and trauma are the primary causes. If the nails are permitted to grow, they may take on the appearance of a horn. This is called onychogryphosis. (Courtesy of Department of Dermatology, UCSD.)

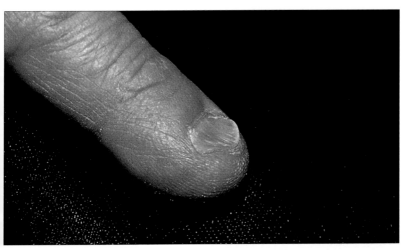

Figure 422. Koilonychia. The nail is concave with the plate thinned and the edges everted in koilonychia, also known as spoon nails. It occurs not uncommonly in children on the hallux and may be familial. Associations include occupational trauma, Plummer–Vinson syndrome, iron deficiency anemia and many others.

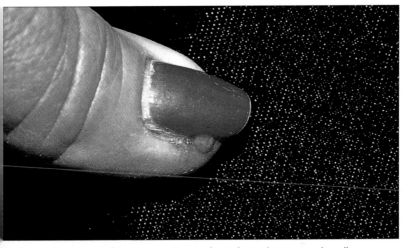

Figure 423. Paronychia, acute. An acutely tender, red, periungual swelling occurs in acute paronychia. Pus may be visible below the cuticle. The nail is usually not dystrophic. *Staphylococcus aureus* or *Streptococcus* are the usual pathogens. Anaerobes and *Candida* may also be found. Risk factors include trauma, manipulation and isotretinoin.

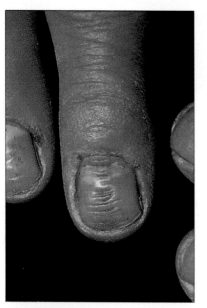

Figure 424. Paronychia, chronic.
The periungual areas of multiple nails are swollen, red and inflamed in chronic paronychia. The cuticle is lost and dystrophy of the nail often occurs. *Candida, Proteus, Klebsiella, Staphylococcus, Pseudomonas* and saprophytic fungi are potential pathogens. Risk factors include manicures, pushing back the cuticle, and frequent contact with water (e.g. housewives, bartenders). Several cases of immediate hypersensitivity to foods in food handlers have been reported to cause a chronic paronychia, as has allergic contact dermatitis to nail polish.

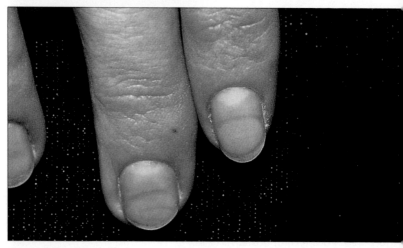

Figure 425. Beau's lines. A transverse furrow or ridge of the nail plate that develops after various diseases or chemotherapy is called a Beau's line. It is caused by temporary arrest of nail plate function. This patient had suffered from infectious mononucleosis four months before presentation.

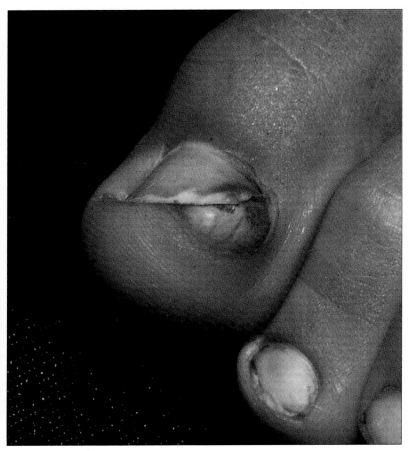

Figure 426. Exostosis. A firm subungual papule or nodule protruding from under the distal nail is characteristic. The dorsal, medial aspect of the hallux is the most common site. Dystrophy of the overlying nail plate may occur. Diagnosis is by X-ray. A benign osseous proliferation is the underlying cause.

See also onychomycosis (**Figure 293**), mucocutaneous candidiasis (**Figure 294**), proximal subungual onychomycosis (**Figure 254**), white superficial onychomycosis (**Figure 255**), acral lentiginous melanoma (**Figure 458**) and Terry's nails (**Figure 563**).

Oral Mucosa

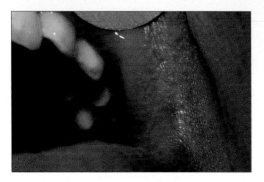

Figure 427. Fordyce spots. These tiny, multiple, pinpoint, yellow papules on the lips or buccal mucosa represent ectopic sebaceous glands and are usually an incidental finding requiring no treatment.

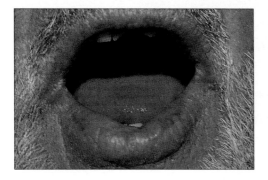

Figure 428. Perleche. Redness, scaling and crusting at the corner of the mouth occur in angular cheilitis, also known as perleche. This disease represents yet another type of intertrigo where body folds opposed keep the skin excessively moist and macerated. Bacteria and *Candida* may cause secondary infection. Lip licking in the young, mouth breathing (day or night or related to orthodontic devices causing excessive saliva) and decreased vertical separation of the mandible and maxilla (e.g. in older patients from lack of teeth or bone resorption) causing a prominent skin fold are all risk factors.

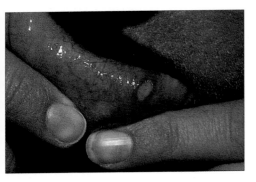

Figure 429. Aphthous ulcer. These shallow intraoral ulcers can be extremely painful and often come in crops. The greyish center is usually surrounded by a bright red halo. Extensive and painful aphthosis may occur in patients with HIV infection. Genital and oral ulceration associated with iritis occurs in Behçet's syndrome (see **Figure 334**).

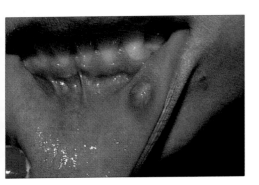

Figure 430. Mucocele. A solitary, translucent, cystic papulonodule on the inner surface of the lip is characteristic. This pseudocyst (no epithelial lining) contains mucin and results from obstruction of the secretory ducts of a salivary gland.

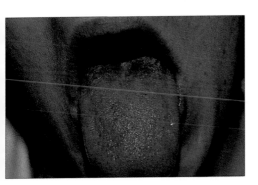

Figure 431. Black hairy tongue. The surface of the tongue is black, velvety and hairlike in this unusual condition. Topical or oral antibiotics, poor oral hygiene, smoking, alcohol or the use of mouthwashes may precipitate this condition.

See also pemphigus vulgaris (**Figure 184**), cicatricial pemphigoid (**Figure 190**), paraneoplastic pemphigus (**Figure 185**), geographic tongue (**Figure 510**), lichen planus (**Figures 517 and 518**).

Photodistributed Disorders

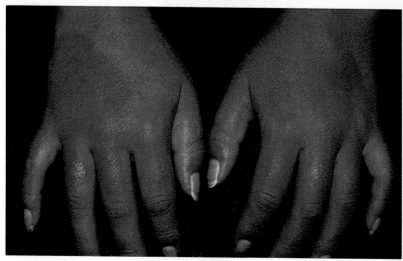

Figure 432. Phytophotocontact dermatitis. Burning, erythema and, if severe, bulla formation followed by dark post-inflammatory hyperpigmentation distributed in bizarre linear arrangements are characteristic. The cause is furocoumarins in plants or fruit, which when inadvertently placed in contact with the skin, make it photosensitive. Common offenders include oranges, limes, lemons, celery, figs, dill, carrots and parsley. This patient squeezed limes in preparing tropical drinks at an outdoor party. (See **Figure 475**.)

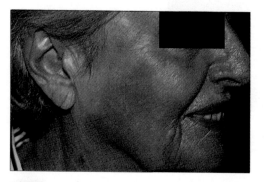

Figure 433. Photoallergic contact dermatitis. This woman's facial erythema resulted from a photocontact reaction with an ingredient in her moisturizer. Sunscreens are currently one of the most common causes of photoallergy. It is believed that ultraviolet light alters the compound, creating an allergen to which the patient is allergic.

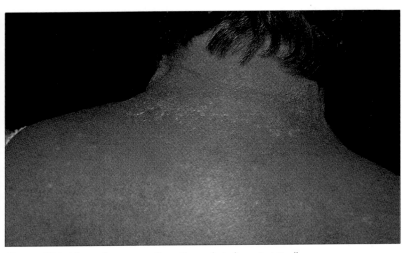

Figure 434. Photodrug eruption. Drugs that characteristically cause photosensitivity include non-steroidal anti-inflammatories, quinacrine (as shown here), doxycycline and thiazides.

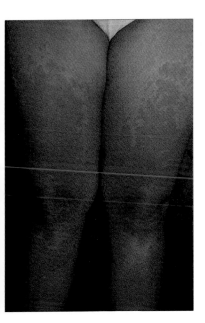

Figure 435. Polymorphous light eruption. Several hours after sun exposure, patients may develop papulovesicular, urticarial, papular or plaque-type lesions. The face and neck are not typically affected as these areas, through regular exposure, harden to the sun's effects. Outbreaks occur in the summer and may affect any photoexposed area. Patients who travel to sun-intense areas for brief vacations may be most severely affected. Antinuclear antibody (ANA) and Ro (SS-A) should be obtained to exclude lupus erythematosus.

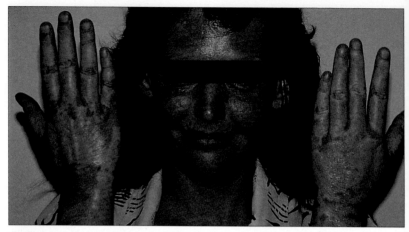

Figure 436. Systemic lupus erythematosus. Several patterns of photosensitivity may occur in lupus erythematosus. Bilateral erythema of the cheeks and malar eminences (butterfly rash) and/or a more extensive photodistributed rash may be seen in systemic lupus erythematosus (SLE) (see also **Figure 194**). Discoid lesions that are more fixed and discrete tend to occur in photoexposed areas such as the face, scalp and upper trunk in both disseminated lupus erythematosus and SLE (see **Figures 196 and 197**). Finally, photodistributed papulosquamous or annular lesions may occur in subacute cutaneous lupus erythematosus (**Figures 199 and 200**)

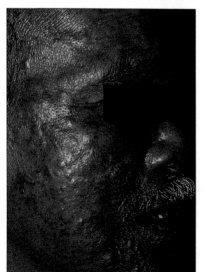

Figure 437. Chronic actinic dermatosis. Persistent erythema of the face in a middle-aged to elderly person is characteristic. With time, the skin may become eczematous and lichenified, and a leonine facies may result. Although histologic features may suggest a lymphoma, chronic actinic dermatosis is not a premalignant condition. For unclear reasons, these patients have a high incidence of contact allergy sensitivity to plant oleoresin extracts, fragrances and lichens.

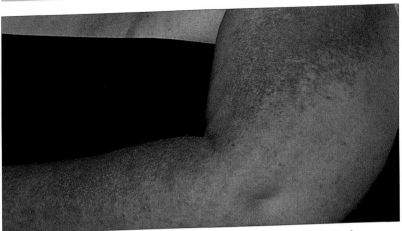

Figure 438. Dermatomyositis. The erythematous rash of dermatomyositis often occurs in a photosensitive distribution, commonly affecting the upper back and chest as well as the photoexposed areas of the arms. Other characteristic changes include periorbital edema and red, scaly papules over the knuckles. (See also **Figures 201 and 202**.)

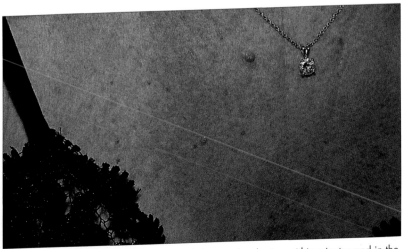

Figure 439. Solar urticaria. Urticarial plaques developing within minutes and in the exact distribution of sun exposure are characteristic of solar urticaria. Systemic symptoms including syncope may occur. The lesions usually resolve within hours. ANA, Ro and La should be negative.

Nevi and Melanoma

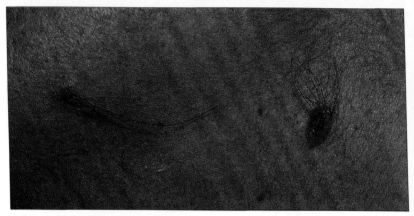

Figure 440. Benign nevus. Common, acquired nevi begin appearing in the first year of life. They grow in size and number peaking in the third or fourth decade. They are most common above the waist on the sun-exposed skin. Significant hair growth may be found as illustrated here.

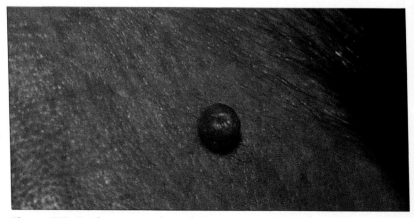

Figure 441. Benign nevus, dermal. Benign nevi may be categorized generally as flat and pigmented (junctional), raised and pigmented (compound) or raised and flesh-colored (dermal).

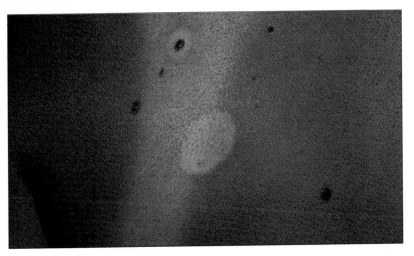

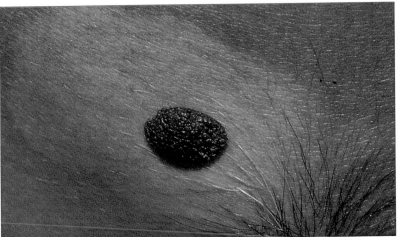

Figures 442 and 443. Halo nevus. The immune system in a child may, for unknown reasons, pick a mole to 'attack'. In the process, a surrounding ring of pigment is lost. Vitiligo may occasionally be found in the same patient. A halo nevus, like any other, should be evaluated by the ABCD (see **Figure 452**) criteria and, if atypical, removed. If left alone, the mole will shrink up and disappear over several years. In **Figure 442**, a halo nevus is seen in the upper middle of the photograph. In the center, a halo is left as its mole has been 'removed' by the immune system. Note also that the right half of this halo is erythematous, being sunburned instead of tanned because of its lack of pigment. Rarely, congenital nevi may develop a halo (**Figure 443**).

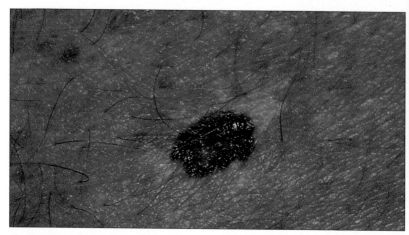

Figure 444. Recurrent nevus. A benign pigmented lesion with atypical clinical and histologic features may develop in the scar of a partially removed nevus. Melanoma, however, must always be considered.

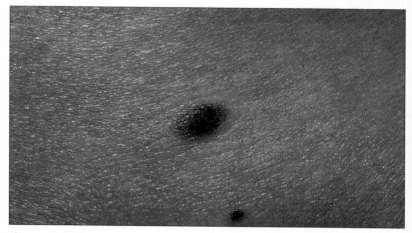

Figure 445. Blue nevus. A small, solitary, round, blue macule or papule on the dorsa of the hands is characteristic of a blue nevus. It may also occur on the scalp or feet. A nodular type occasionally occurs on the buttocks. The brown pigment of the dermis looks blue because of the Tyndall effect.

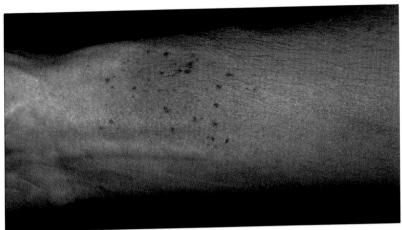

Figure 446. Nevus spilus. A tan patch speckled with brown or black spots is typical. Onset is usually in childhood or adolescence. Lesions are typically 1–5 cm in size but rarely may be much larger. In some lesions, the background tan color is absent. Very rarely, malignant change may occur.

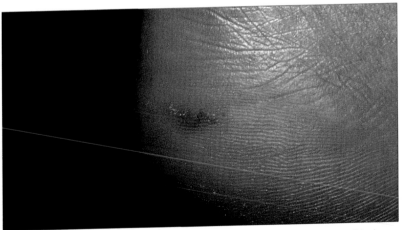

Figure 447. Talon noire. Talon noire or black heel is characterized by tiny black pinpoint dots grouped together and located somewhere along the posterior edge of the heel. The patients are usually athletically involved in sports such as basketball, soccer, volleyball, etc. Sheer forces causing extravasation of blood are thought to be the cause. The lesion is most commonly confused with a verruca and occasionally a melanoma. A similar change may occur on the palmar aspect of the fingers.

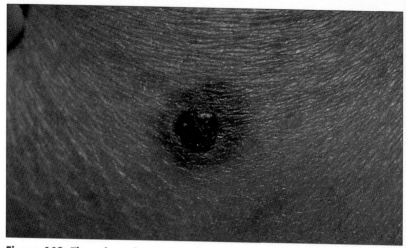

Figure 448. Thrombosed angiokeratoma. A solitary angiokeratoma may thrombose, with the resultant lesion resembling a melanoma.

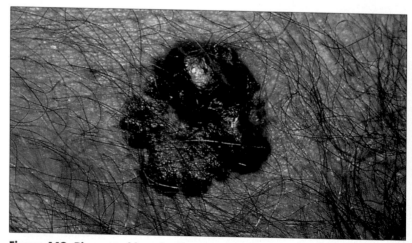

Figure 449. Pigmented basal cell carcinoma. Occasionally, a basal cell carcinoma may retain enough pigment to mimic a melanoma.(See also **Figure 600**.) (Courtesy of Department of Dermatology, UCSD.)

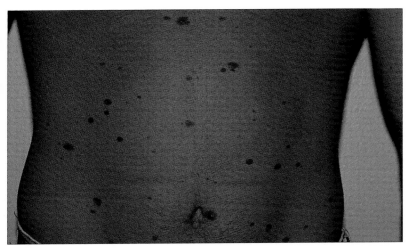

Figure 450. Familial atypical mole–melanoma syndrome. The familial atypical mole–melanoma syndrome (FAM–M syndrome) combines a personal or family history of melanoma with multiple clinically atypical nevi. These patients often have a large number of nevi (e.g. > 50) as well as nevi in unusual sites, e.g. the buttocks, dorsa of the feet, anterior aspect of the scalp, etc. Patients should be monitored closely as their risk for developing melanoma is high.

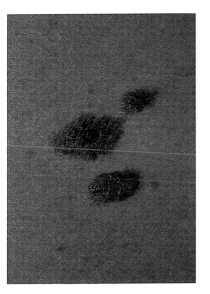

Figure 451. Familial atypical mole–melanoma syndrome. Close-up examination shows nevi with irregular borders, diameter > 6 mm and irregular colors.

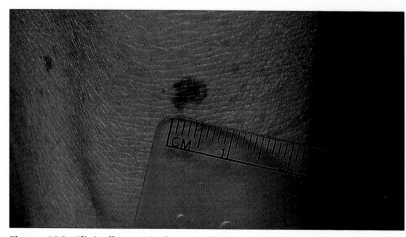

Figure 452. Clinically atypical nevus, benign. Every new dermatologic patient should be encouraged to have a complete skin examination. Return patients should have one every 2–3 years. Monthly self-examination should also be encouraged. All pigmented lesions should be evaluated by the ABCD criteria. Any lesion with two of the following should be termed a clinically atypical nevus and removed for histologic examination: i) **a**symmetric shape, ii) irregular **b**order, iii) variegated **c**olor and iv) **d**iameter greater than 6 mm. Although irregular in shape and containing multiple colors, this lesion was benign.

Figure 453. Clinically atypical nevus—melanoma *in situ*. If the lesion fulfils the histologic criteria for melanoma but is confined to the epidermis, the term melanoma *in situ* is used. At this initial stage, there is no possibility of metastatic spread.

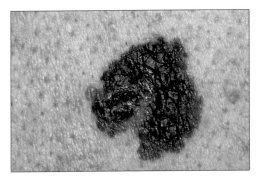

Figure 454. Melanoma, superficial spreading. All the ABCD criteria are fulfilled here. The lesion is large, irregular in shape, border and color. Risk factors for melanoma include the presence of one or more of the following: clinically atypical (formerly called dysplastic) nevi, increased number of nevi, family history of melanoma, increased propensity to sunburn, a tendency to freckle and blond or red hair.

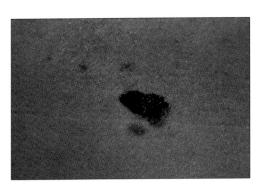

Figure 455. Melanoma. Melanomas may arise from normal skin or from a pre-existing nevus as shown here.

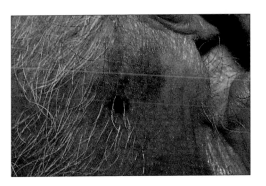

Figure 456. Lentigo maligna melanoma. A slowly enlarging, irregularly pigmented, irregularly shaped macule on the sun-exposed skin of an older adult is characteristic. A Wood's light may be helpful in delineating the extent of the lesion. Histologically, lentigo maligna remains confined to the epidermis. When invasion into the dermis occurs, the term lentigo maligna melanoma is used.

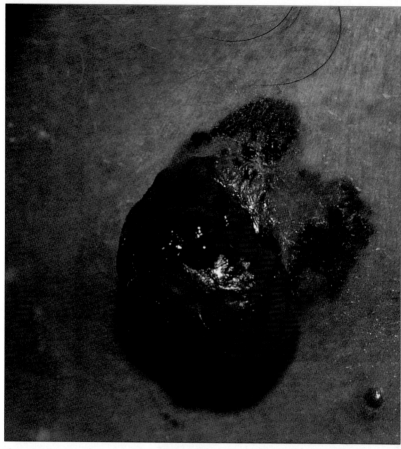

Figure 457. Nodular melanoma. A melanoma may occasionally present as a rapidly growing nodule. It may be brown or black or relatively devoid of pigment, as shown here. Any focus of pigment within a vascular lesion should arouse suspicion.

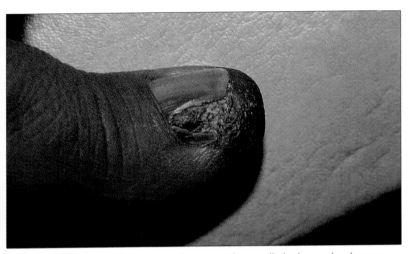

Figure 458. Acral lentiginous melanoma. The so-called subungual melanoma probably begins in the nail matrix and presents initially as longitudinal melanonychia (see **Figure 419**). As the melanoma spreads, nail destruction may occur with pigment extending to the proximal nail fold (Hutchison's sign) or to the fingertip.

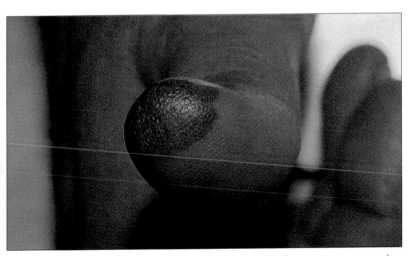

Figure 459. Acral lentiginous melanoma. Rarely, a melanoma may occur on the palms, soles, fingers or toes. When Black patients develop melanoma, this is the most common type.

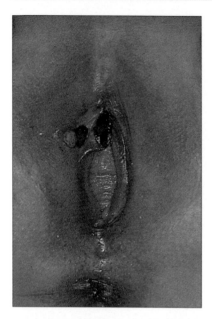

Figure 460. Melanoma, vulva.
Benign nevi, vulvar melanosis and melanoma may occur in the vulvar region. Any pigmented lesion should be evaluated for irregularity in shape or color and biopsied if indicated. The patient shown developed her melanoma at 75 years of age. (Courtesy of Paul Koonings, MD.)

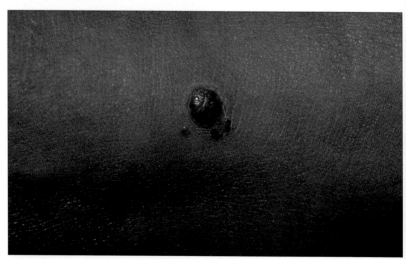

Figure 461. Amelanotic melanoma. Rarely, melanomas may be totally devoid of pigment, making the diagnosis very difficult. This vascular papule on the ankle of a 22-year-old woman was thought to be a hemangioma.

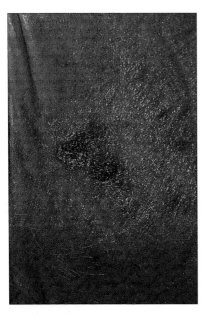

Figure 462. Amelanotic lentigo maligna. In very rare cases, a lentigo maligna may be devoid of pigment. The correct diagnosis is rarely suspected. This red scaly lesion was thought to represent Bowen's disease or a basal cell carcinoma. Only after two biopsies was the correct diagnosis believed.

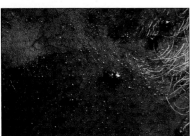

Figure 463. Metastatic melanoma, pigmented. Melanomas may recur at the surgical site, in transit to regional lymph nodes or at distant sites. Multiple pigmented cutaneous lesions may occur as shown. Diffuse hyperpigmentation and melanuria can develop rarely. (Photograph courtesy of Department of Dermatology, UCSD.)

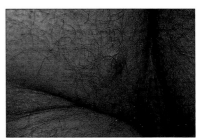

Figure 464. Metastatic melanoma, red. Any new cutaneous growth in a patient with a history of melanoma should be considered as a possible metastatic focus. This new erythematous papule of the left buttocks represented metastatic melanoma.

See also spitz nevus (**Figure 101**).

Pigmentary Disorders

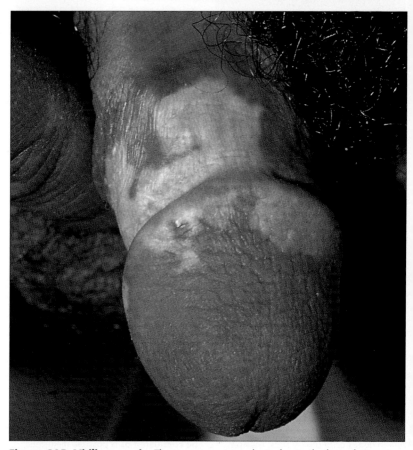

Figure 465. Vitiligo, penis. The immune system selectively attacks the melanin-producing cells of the skin in vitiligo. Sharply depigmented, often symmetric patches occurring anywhere but with preference for the face, fingers, trunk and extremities, result. Peak onset is 10–30 years of age. Patients with onset over 40 years of age should have a complete skin examination to exclude coexistent melanoma. Various autoimmune diseases are associated, with demonstration of autoantibodies typical (e.g. thyroid). A chemical leukoderma from industrial exposure to hydroquinones, catechols, phenols or mercaptoamines is rare but occurs and can be indistinguishable from vitiligo.

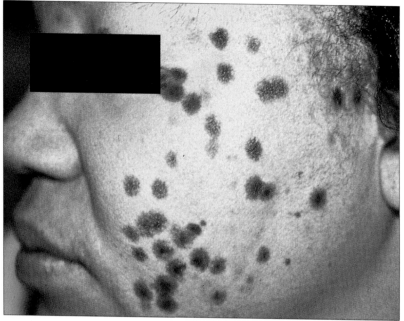

Figure 466. Vitiligo, diffuse. Such diffuse loss of pigmentation can be psychologically devastating. (Courtesy of Theodore Sebastian, MD.)

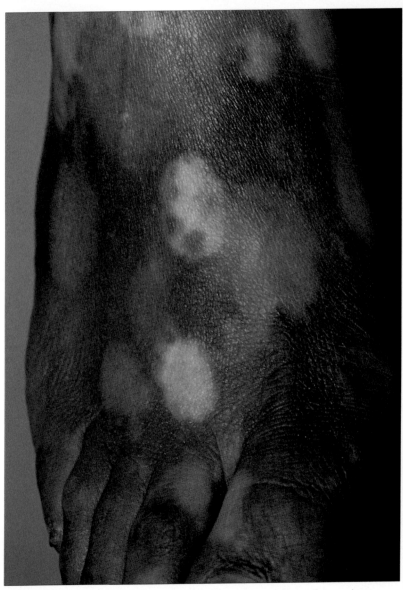

Figure 467. Trichrome vitiligo. Occasionally, an intermediate color may be present making the patient 'three-colored'.

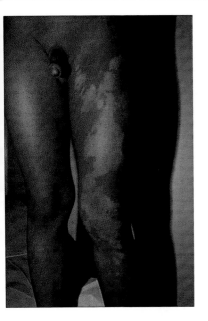

Figure 468. Segmental vitiligo. In this distinct variant of vitiligo, an acquired depigmented patch of skin in a segmental or dermatomal pattern occurs. In contrast to the typical vitiligo, new lesions cease after 1 year, onset is in childhood in the majority, Koebnerization does not occur, halo nevi are not associated and response to Psoralen plus ultraviolet light photochemotherapy is poor. (Courtesy of Michael O Murphy, MD.)

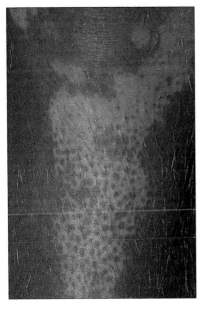

Figure 469. Follicular repigmentation of vitiligo. When vitiligo repigments, it often does so initially about the hair follicles.

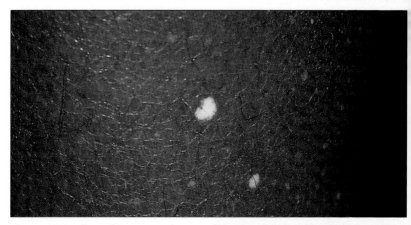

Figure 470. Idiopathic guttate hypomelanosis. Multiple, white macules, usually 1–4 mm in diameter symmetrically distributed on the outer forearms or extensor legs are characteristic. Women are more commonly affected than men, as are people over 40 years of age. The cause is unknown.

See also post-inflammatory hypopigmentation (**Figure 178**), steroid hypopigmentation (**Figure 179**) and halo nevi (**Figures 442 and 443**).

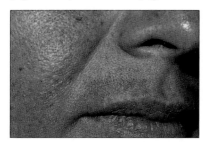

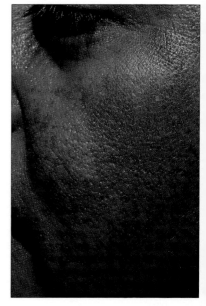

Figures 471(above) **and 472** (right). **Melasma.** The combination of female hormones (e.g. pregnancy, oral contraceptives) and the sun combine to cause this disease. Symmetric, uniformly hyperpigmented, sharply defined macules and patches on the face in the sun-exposed areas of a woman result. It commonly affects the upper lip, cheeks and forehead. Although both sexes and all races may be affected, women with darker skin predominate.

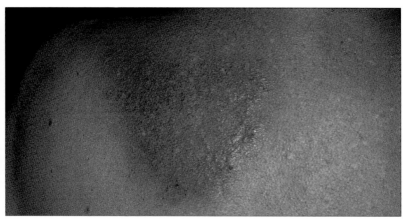

Figure 473. Macular amyloidosis, back. Dark brown patches that may have a reticulated or rippled pattern on the upper back, usually to one side, occur in macular amyloidosis. Middle-aged, dark-skinned patients are commonly affected. A habit of scratching is often found and may be carried out with a variety of instruments including the fingers, back scratchers, towels or a nylon brush. The amyloid in this instance is derived from keratinocytes.

Figure 474. Macular amyloidosis, shins. Note the uniformity of the color and the rippled pattern.

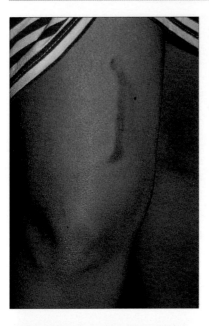

Figure 475. Phytophotocontact dermatitis. Burning, erythema and, when severe, bulla formation, followed by dark post-inflammatory hyper-pigmentation distributed in bizarre linear arrangements are characteristic. (See also **Figure 432**.)

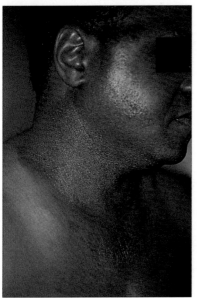

Figure 476. Post-inflammatory hyperpigmentation. Dark patches may develop after almost any disturbance of the skin in a dark-skinned patient. This patient had experienced an allergic contact dermatitis to a cologne. (Courtesy of Steven Goldberg, MD.)

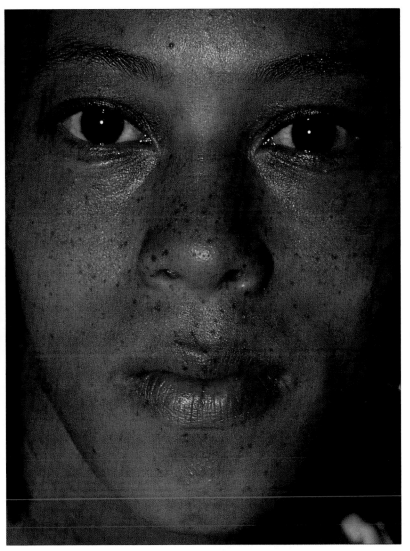

Figure 477. Patterned inherited lentiginosis. This patient with patterned inherited lentiginosis has a striking lentiginous pigmentation of the central face and lips without mucous membrane or internal involvement. Lentigines may also be seen elsewhere, e.g. the buttocks or elbows. Inheritance is autosomal dominant. No systemic abnormalities are associated. Darker-skinned patients are most commonly affected.

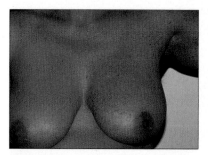

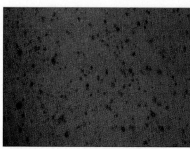

Figure 478. Agminated lentiginosis. In this condition, multiple pigmented macules are distributed in a quasi-dermatomal pattern. This woman's left arm, axilla and breast were affected.

Figure 479. Leopard syndrome. This mnemonic stands for **l**entigines, **e**lectrocardiogram abnormalities, **o**cular hypertelorism, **p**ulmonary stenosis, **a**bnormal genitalia, **r**etardation of growth and **d**eafness. The darkly pigmented freckles or lentigines begin in infancy and progress. An autosomal dominant inheritance pattern occurs. Only some of the non-cutaneous findings may be present in any one patient. An electrocardiogram should always be obtained.

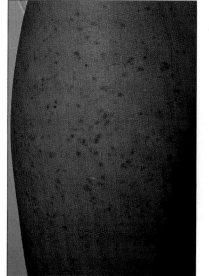

Figure 480. Urticaria pigmentosa. Various patterns of cutaneous mastocytosis occur. In urticaria pigmentosa, multiple, brown macules or papules occur scattered on the body. Patients may have a few to several thousand. The pigmentation histologically is basal melanosis. See also **Figures 98–100**.

(See also Peutz–Jeghers syndrome, **Figure 57**).

Pregnancy-Related Dermatoses

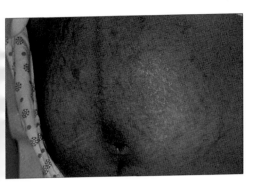

Figure 481. Linea nigra.
A linear streak running vertically along the midline of the abdomen from the symphysis pubis to the xyphoid process occurring in pregnancy is characteristic of linea nigra. Striae distensae, which commonly develop in pregnancy are also shown.

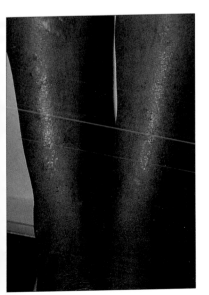

Figure 482. Pruritus in pregnancy.
A significant percentage of pregnant women may develop pruritus during pregnancy. One must always rule out non-pregnancy-related causes such as scabies, xerosis, atopic dermatitis, etc. Potential pregnancy-related causes include cholestasis and early pemphigoid gestationis. The majority, however, fall into a broad and poorly defined category, as did this patient. Most of her skin changes are from scratching.

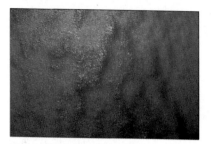

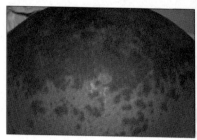

Figure 483. Pruritic urticarial papules and plaques of pregnancy. PUPPP occurs principally in primigravidas in the third trimester. Urticarial, papular and polycyclic lesions classically begin in the abdominal stria (as shown here) and abdomen but then may spread to the trunk, arms, thighs and buttocks. PUPPP does not routinely flare postpartum as does herpes gestationis and has no tendency to recur in subsequent pregnancies. Direct immunofluorescence is negative. (Courtesy of Steven Goldberg, MD.)

Figure 484. PUPPP. Urticarial plaques occurred predominantly in this patient. (Courtesy of Michael O Murphy, MD.)

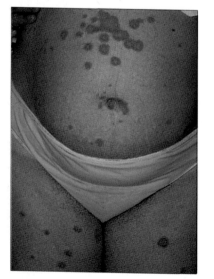

Figure 485. Pemphigoid gestationis, urticarial plaques. The skin lesions of pemphigoid gestationis (also known as herpes gestationis) often begin on the abdomen and include urticarial plaques and vesicles. Onset is usually in the second and third trimester but may occur in the first trimester or immediately postpartum. The neonate has skin lesions approximately 5–10% of the time. Despite the name herpes gestationis, this rare pruritic subepidermal bullous eruption of pregnancy is unrelated to any viral infection. Instead, it represents an autoimmune attack on the skin.

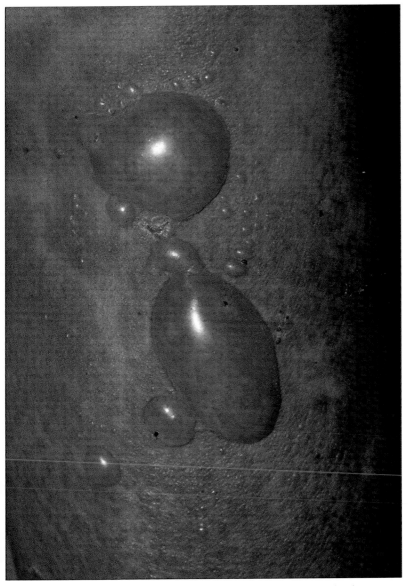

Figure 486. Pemphigoid gestationis, bulla Large bulla may later develop, as in this patient who was experiencing a postpartum flare.

Figure 487. Impetigo herpetiformis This disease has been called pustular psoriasis of pregnancy because of its clinical and histological resemblance to psoriasis, although no personal or family history of psoriasis is usually found. Superficial pustules studded on the periphery of erythematous plaques are characteristic. Hypocalcemia may be a precipitating factor, with tetany and convulsions. Stillbirths, placental insufficiency and perinatal death are associated fetal complications.

See also spider angioma (**Figure 87**) and telogen effluvium (**Figure 239**).

Psoriasis, Lichen Planus and Related Disorders

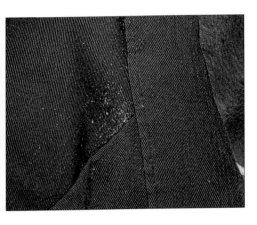

Figure 488. Dandruff. The term dandruff applies to excessive scaling of the scalp. Pruritus is common. Inflammation and erythema are absent. Anyone will develop this condition if they shampoo infrequently enough.

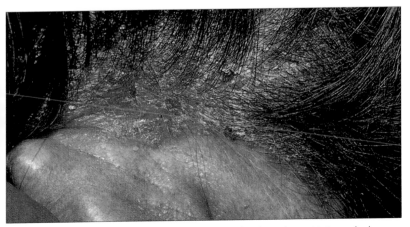

Figure 489. Seborrheic dermatitis. The term seborrheic dermatitis is used when some degree of inflammation and erythema is associated with scale in the seborrheic areas, that is the scalp, face and trunk. The hair itself is unaffected. Overgrowth of the lipophilic yeast *Pityrosporum ovale* has been hypothesized as the etiologic agent.

255

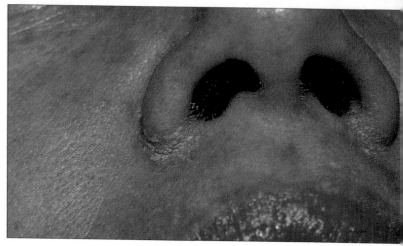

Figure 490. Seborrheic dermatitis, perinasal. Seborrheic dermatitis not only affects the scalp, but also the eyebrows, nasolabial folds and midchest. Significant redness and scale of the nasolabial folds are seen here.

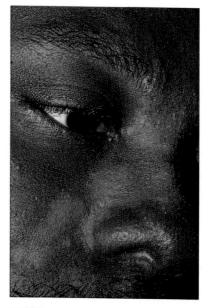

Figure 491. Seborrheic dermatitis. Seborrheic dermatitis is more common in Black patients because they tend to shampoo infrequently. Significant post-inflammatory hypopigmentation may occur.

Figure 492. Seborrheic dermatitis. Annular forms may occur.

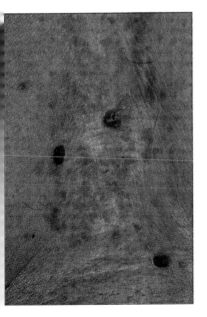

Figure 493. Seborrheic dermatitis, chest. The red, scaly midchest in this adult man is typical of seborrheic dermatitis.

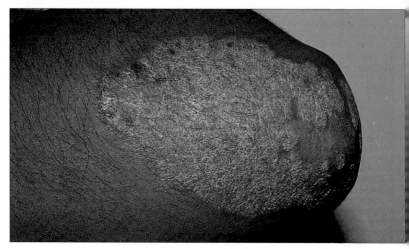

Figure 494. Psoriasis, papulosquamous plaque. Psoriasis affects 1–2% of the population. The classic lesion is a sharply demarcated, raised, red plaque, covered with silvery-white scale. The elbows, knees, scalp and intergluteal cleft are frequently involved. Koebnerization is typical. The disease tends to be chronic with periodic flares.

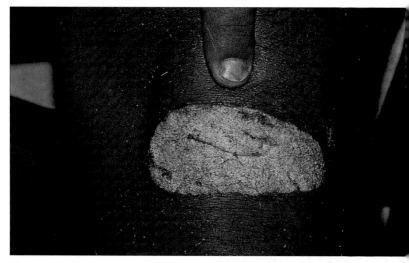

Figure 495. Psoriasis, papulosquamous plaque. A familial tendency is typical but other factors are also involved. Various drugs (e.g. beta-blockers), stress or a streptococcal infection may precipitate a flare.

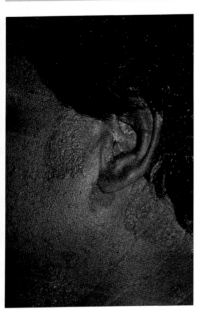

Figure 496. Psoriasis, scalp. Scalp psoriasis—like seborrheic dermatitis—manifests itself as redness and scaling of the scalp. However, the crust is thicker, the lesions are more well-defined and they are often more resistant to treatment. A plaque of redness and scale encircling the scalp, extending 1–2 cm beyond the hair line, is also characteristic and is shown here.

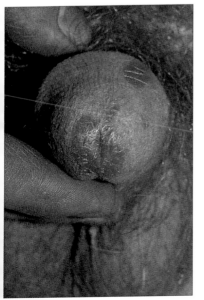

Figure 497. Psoriasis, penis. The genitalia of both men and women are commonly involved.

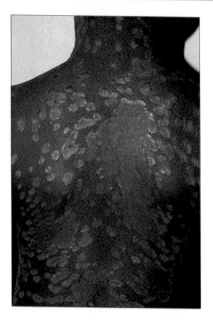

Figure 498. Psoriasis, Black child.
Psoriasis in a Black patient often leads to significant post-inflammatory hypopigmentation, as shown here.

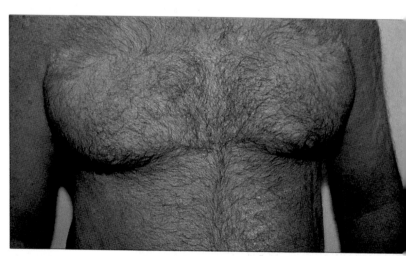

Figure 499. Psoriasis, diffuse. Psoriasis may spread to cover most of the body. The extent of involvement is usually measured by calculating the percentage of total body surface area affected.

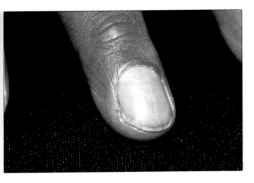

Figure 500. Psoriasis, nail pitting. Approximately half of patients with psoriasis may show nail involvement. When the matrix is involved, pits may form as shown here.

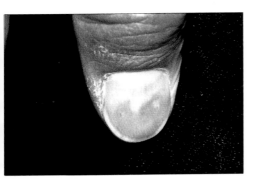

Figure 501. Psoriasis, oil spot. A yellow–brown subungual discoloration in a patient with psoriasis indicates involvement of the nail bed.

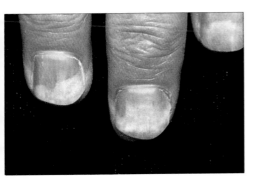

Figure 502. Psoriasis, onycholysis. If the nail bed is affected, onycholysis (separation of the nail plate from the bed) may occur.

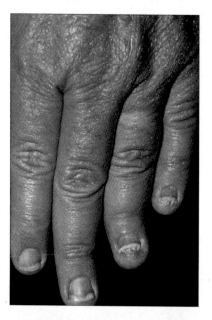

Figure 503. Psoriasis, psoriatic arthropathy. Various forms of seronegative arthritis occur in patients with psoriasis. The joints of the hands and fingers are most frequently involved often with nail damage, as shown here. Severe bone and joint destruction may occur.

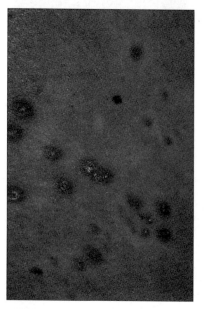

Figure 504. Psoriasis, guttate type. The sudden development of disseminated 0.5–2.0 cm, red, scaly papules or small plaques is characteristic of acute, guttate (drop-shaped) psoriasis. A streptococcal infection is a very common precipitant. Children with psoriasis most often have this form. Spontaneous remission may occur or the disease may evolve into chronic plaque-type psoriasis. (See also **Figures 118 and 119**.)

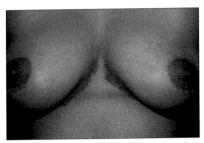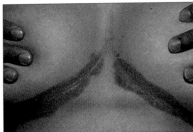

Figures 505 (left) **and 506** (right). **Psoriasis, infra-mammary.** Inverse psoriasis is a term that applies to psoriasis of the body folds. The axilla, inframmary area, gluteal cleft and inguinal crease may be affected. Because of the moist, hydrated environment, scale is usually absent.

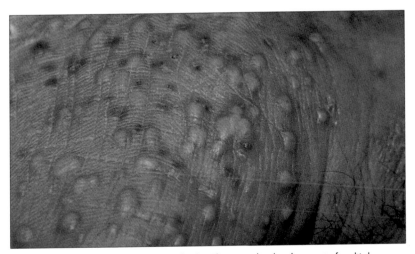

Figure 507. Palmoplantar pustulosis. The periodic development of multiple pustules on the palms and/or soles is characteristic. Often the pustules do not rupture but instead turn brown. The course is chronic. An arthrosteitis has been associated and may be manifested by painful episodes of the anterior chest wall and, less commonly, the knee, spine and ankle. Smoking is strongly associated.

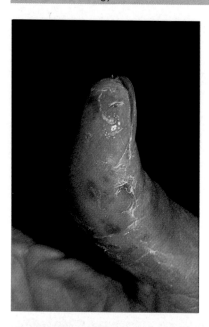

Figure 508. Acrodermatitis continua of Hallopeau. Sterile pustules on one or more fingers and fingertips that rupture leaving tender, eroded skin are characteristic. In the chronic stages, the skin may take on a papulosquamous appearance.

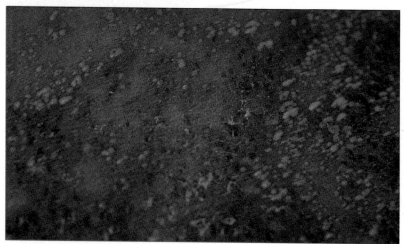

Figure 509. Psoriasis, pustular. In generalized pustular psoriasis of von Zumbusch, fever, generalized erythema and pustules develop acutely. Erythematous plaques with pustules at the periphery are also characteristic. Hypoalbuminemia, hypocalcemia, loss of intravascular fluid and renal failure are potential complications.

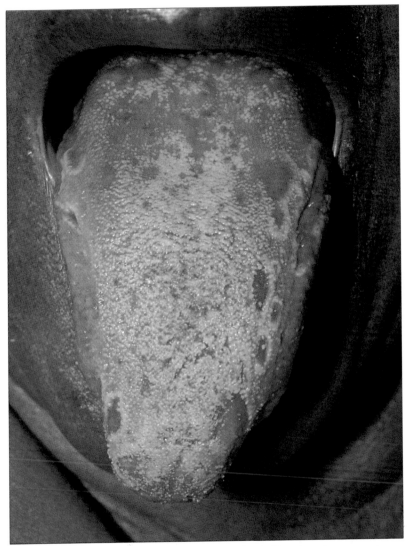

Figure 510. Geographic tongue. Smooth atrophic 'bald' red patches or annular, serpiginous, white, yellow lines occur in geographic tongue, also known as benign migratory glossitis or glossitis areata migrans. Combinations of the two forms occur. This condition is 4–5 times more prevalent in psoriatic patients and may occur anywhere in the mouth.

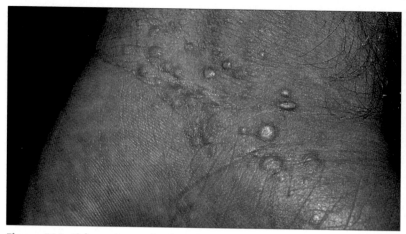

Figure 511. Lichen planus. Purple, polygonal, flat-topped papules often on the inner wrists, penis, periorbital area, soles and trunk occur in lichen planus. A white, lace-like appearance of the surface (Wickham's striae) is characteristic. Patients with chronic liver disease (e.g. primary biliary cirrhosis, chronic active hepatitis) have twice the risk of developing lichen planus compared with the general population. Some of these patients are infected with hepatitis B and some with hepatitis C.

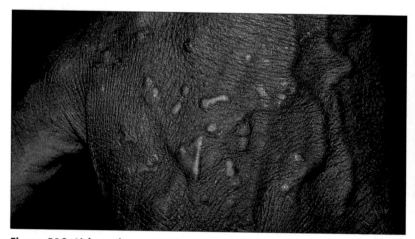

Figure 512. Lichen planus, Koebner. Lichen planus may occur in areas of trauma. This manual laborer developed several linear lesions on the back of the hands. Note the unique violaceous color that is virtually pathognomonic of lichen planus.

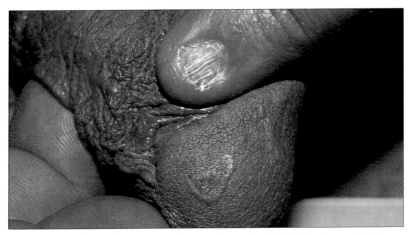

Figure 513. Lichen planus, annular, penis and nail. Nail involvement in lichen planus may take many forms including longitudinal ridging, thinning, onycholysis and pterygium formation. Pterygium is a term used to describe adhesion of the proximal nail plate to the matrix that may cause significant thinning or absence of the nail. Annular lichen planus, as shown here on the penis, has a predilection for the male genitalia. Lichen planus of the penis may also present as purple papules covered by lace-like Wickham's striae.

Figure 514. Lichen planus, papulosquamous. On occasion, lichen planus lesions may develop enough scale to put them in the papulosquamous category.

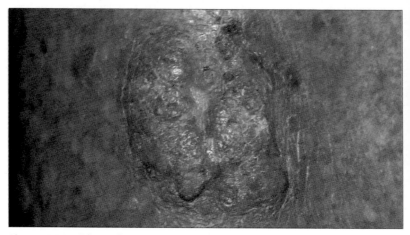

Figure 515. Lichen planus, hypertrophic. Lichen planus may occasionally present as hyperkeratotic nodules or plaques, especially on the legs.

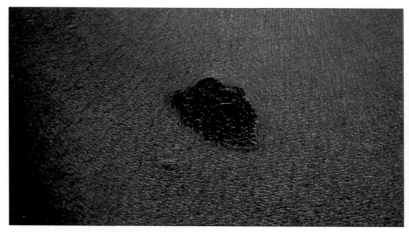

Figure 516. Lichen planus, annular, hyperpigmented. In lichen planus, there is a tremendous attack on the basal layer of the epidermis. Significant deposition of pigment in the dermis may result. This slowly expanding annular lesion of lichen planus is leaving post-inflammatory hyperpigmentation in its wake.

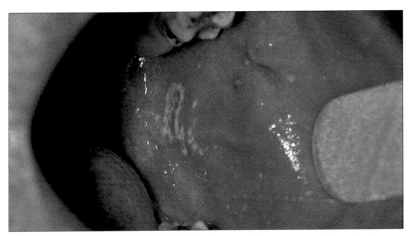

Figure 517. Lichen planus, buccal mucosa. A white, reticulated, lace-like lesion on the buccal mucosa, often bilateral, occurs in lichen planus. This mucosal change is so characteristic of lichen planus that it should be looked for to confirm the diagnosis of lichen planus in atypical cases. Lesions may occur on the tongue and lips as well. It usually is asymptomatic, requiring no treatment.

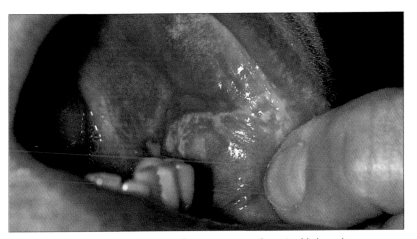

Figure 518. Lichen planus, buccal mucosa, erosive. Oral lichen planus may occasionally erode the mucosa, leading to painful ulcerations. In women, similar changes on the vulvar mucosa may occur. Painful lesions and adhesions can hinder or even prevent intercourse. Rarely, squamous cell carcinoma can arise in either oral or vulvar lichen planus.

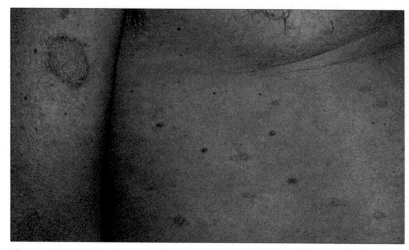

Figure 519. Pityriasis rosea. Pityriasis rosea is a common, diffuse and self-limiting papulosquamous eruption that tends to affect teenagers and young adults. A larger 'herald' patch which predates the more diffuse eruption by 1–3 weeks usually occurs and is shown here on the right arm. Scattered on the trunk are the multiple, oval, red, reasonably well-defined, 1–2 cm plaques with scale. Without the herald patch or other classic features, a rapid plasma reagin should be obtained to rule out secondary syphilis. The rash usually appears over 3 weeks, stays around for 3 weeks and goes away over 3 weeks, although a variant, called chronic pityriasis rosea, may persist.

Figure 520. Pityriasis rosea, incipient. The lesions of pityriasis rosea begin as small erythematous papules, as shown here. The correct diagnosis is rarely made at this stage, unless the herald patch is present. If a patient presents early with only the herald patch, the doctor may incorrectly diagnose ringworm, psoriasis or eczema.

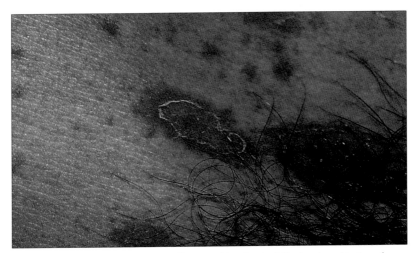

Figure 521. Pityriasis rosea, collarette. The classic, fully developed lesion of pityriasis rosea possesses a peripheral collarette of scale.

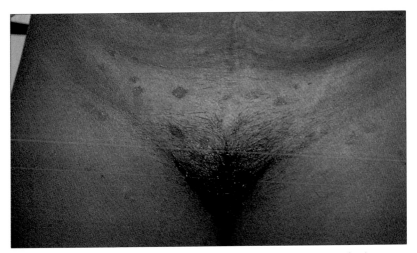

Figure 522. Pityriasis rosea, groin. The lesions of pityriasis rosea prefer the groin and axilla. Occasionally, patients may present with lesions only in these areas. Pityriasis rosea does not like the sun and, in fact, increased sun exposure is one form of treatment.

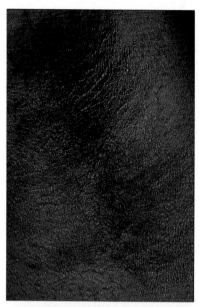

Figure 523. Pityriasis rosea, axilla. The axilla is another classic place for pityriasis rosea to occur. Lesions may be confluent, as shown here. In the dark-skinned patient, a violaceous hue may be present.

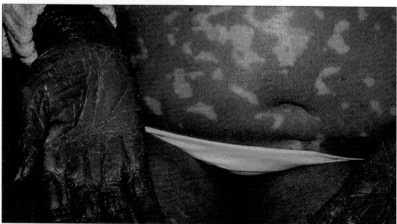

Figure 524. Pityriasis rubra pilaris. Pityriasis rubra pilaris is a rare chronic papulosquamous disease that is characterized by diffuse erythema about islands of sparing (normal skin) and diffuse hyperkeratosis of the palms and soles. Dramatic follicular plugging may occur on the dorsa of the hands and fingers, like a nutmeg grater. Nail pits are usually absent (compared with psoriasis). The redness and scale of pityriasis rubra pilaris often begin on the scalp and progress downward.

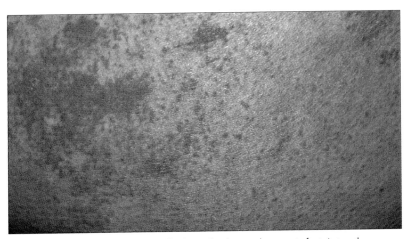

Figure 525. Pityriasis rubra pilaris. Follicular involvement is first. Later, these small orangish-red papules merge to form large plaques.

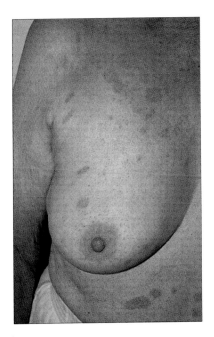

Figure 526. Parapsoriasis, small plaque. The term parapsoriasis refers to chronic papulosquamous lesions in an adult that do not fit the clinical picture of psoriasis. Notably, there is a lack of preference for the elbows, knees, scalp or nails. Parapsoriasis has been broadly divided into small (< 5 cm) and large plaques.

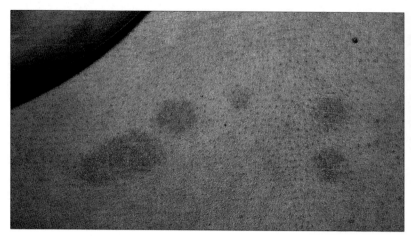

Figure 527. Parapsoriasis, small plaque. Reddish-brown, round to oval, scaly plaques on the trunk that may last years to decades are characteristic of small plaque psoriasis. Elongated or digitate forms occur. Small plaque psoriasis is characteristically non-pruritic. It is generally true that progression to lymphoma does not occur, although pragmatically speaking, persistent disease should be periodically biopsied.

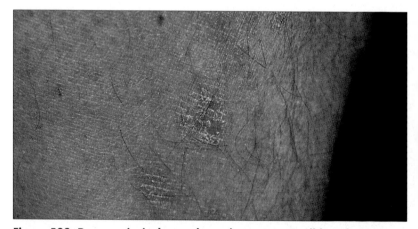

Figure 528. Parapsoriasis, large plaque/cutaneous T-cell lymphoma. Large plaque parapsoriasis is viewed by most as a precursor to cutaneous T-cell lymphoma (CTCL). It may begin insidiously as chronic, fixed, red, scaly lesions on the legs, as shown here. The patient is usually thought to have eczema and may be treated with topical steroids for years. Histologic examination off topical steroids should be repeated at regular intervals until the diagnosis is confirmed.

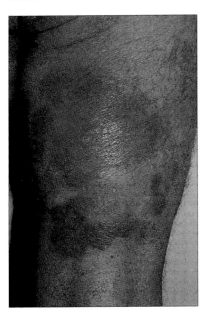

Figure 529. Cutaneous T-cell lymphoma. In CTCL, also known as mycosis fungoides, red, scaly areas develop initially and are followed by infiltrated plaques, figurate lesions and nodules. The sun-protected areas like the buttocks, thighs or legs are favored and lesions are fixed in contrast to eczema.

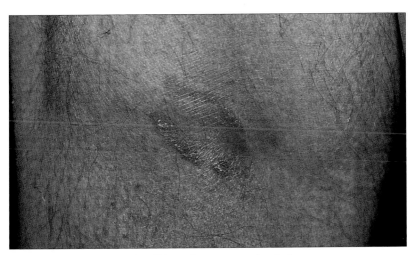

Figure 530. Cutaneous T-cell lymphoma, annular lesion.

Figure 531. Cutaneous T-cell lymphoma, plaque stage. Indurated, dermal papules may coalesce to form large plaques as shown here. Scale may be completely absent.

Figure 532. Cutaneous T-cell lymphoma, poikiloderma. Cutaneous atrophy with prominent telangiectasias is yet another clinical presentation of CTCL.

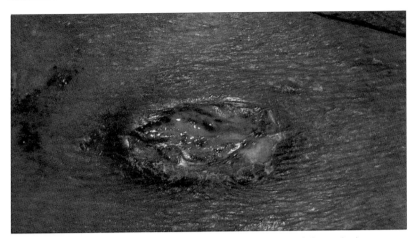

Figure 533. Cutaneous T-cell lymphoma, ulcerative nodule. In the later stages, nodules may develop. They can ulcerate, as shown here. Prognosis is unfavorable if tumors, lymphadenopathy or skin involvement by infiltrated plaques greater than 10% of body surface area are present.

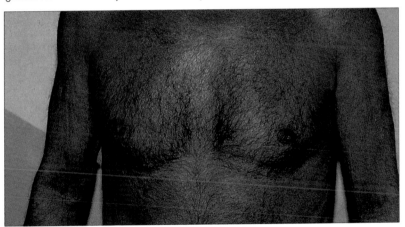

Figure 534. Cutaneous T-cell lymphoma, erythroderma. The adult with diffuse erythroderma may have erythrodermic CTCL. It can develop *de novo* or as a progression of more typical CTCL. The disease may rapidly progress to involve the lymph nodes and blood or it may progress slowly over years. The Sézary syndrome is the triad of generalized erythroderma, lymphadenopathy and atypical mononuclear cells in the peripheral blood.

For related disease, see also PLEVA (**Figure 121**).

Skin Manifestations of Systemic Disease

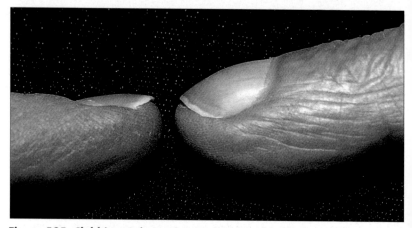

Figure 535. Clubbing. Soft tissue hypertrophy of the distal finger, increased curvature of the nail and a spongy sensation when the base of the nail is compressed are characteristic. Clubbing may occur as a hereditary, isolated finding, associated with congenital cyanotic heart disease, in thyroid acropachy or in association with hypertrophic osteoarthropathy (periosteal new bone formation, painful swelling of the distal extremities, arthritis and malignancy, e.g. bronchogenic carcinoma).

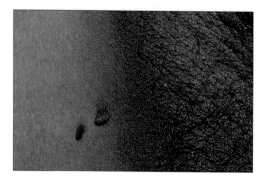

Figure 536. Acanthosis nigricans, neck. A brown, velvety thickening of the skin on the neck, elbows and dorsa of the hands occurs in acanthosis nigricans. It may be familial or associated with obesity or diabetes. (See also **Figure 557**.) Two tags are also seen.

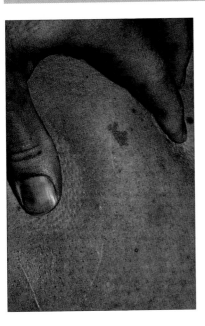

Figure 537. Scleredema diabeticorum. Firm, non-pitting edema of the upper back, often in the shape of an inverted triangle, is characteristic of scleredema diabeticorum and is common in middle-aged, obese, long-standing patients with diabetes. This change is usually better felt than seen.

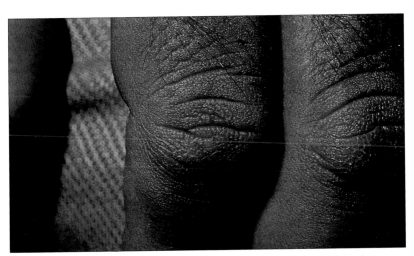

Figure 538. Diabetic finger pebbles. A papillomatous thickening of the skin overlying the knuckles in diabetic patients has been called diabetic finger pebbles.

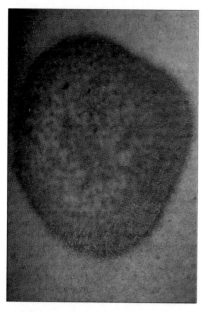

Figure 539. Necrobiosis lipoidica.
Well-demarcated, yellow–red plaques,
with epidermal atrophy on the shins of a
diabetic patient, are characteristic.
Initially, a red plaque forms. As it spreads,
the center becomes depressed and yellow
with telangiectasias. Lesions may occur
elsewhere and may be unassociated with
diabetes.

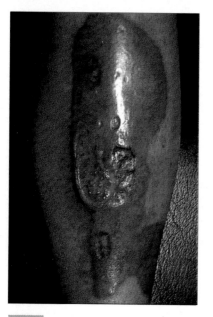

**Figure 540. Necrobiosis lipoidica,
late, ulcerative.** Ulceration is not
uncommon in well-developed lesions.
(Courtesy of Michael O Murphy, MD.)

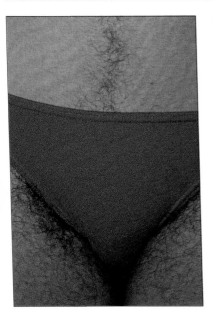

Figure 541. Hirsutism. Excessive terminal hair is seen on the upper lip, cheeks and chin in a woman with hirsutism. The breasts, lower abdomen and elsewhere may also be affected. Hirsutism is more common in women of Eurasian descent. Laboratory evaluation may include dehydroepiandrosterone-sulfate, testosterone and prolactin. These are usually normal however. When signs of virilization are present (e.g. deep voice, clitoral hypertrophy, hair loss), the presence of a hormone-secreting tumor should be considered. (See also **Figure 142**.)

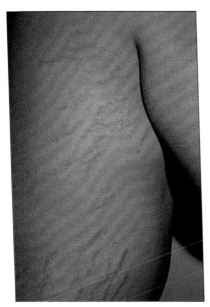

Figure 542. Striae distensae. Striae are common during adolescence, rapid weight gain and during pregnancy. They may also follow potent topical steroid use and Cushing's disease. Initially, they are red/purple and eventually fade to leave thin silvery scars.

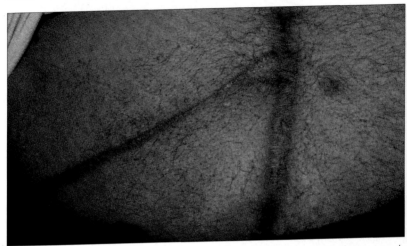

Figure 543. Addisonian pigmentation. Darker pigmentation of the photoexposed skin, of the nipples and areola, of scars (as shown here), the oral mucosa, the periorbital and anogenital areas may occur in patients with adrenocortical insufficiency or Addison's disease.

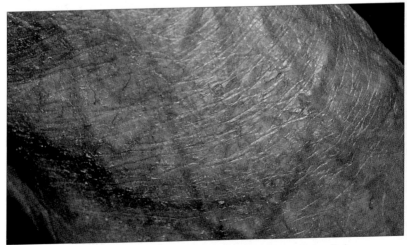

Figure 544. Hypothyroidism. Dry, coarse, cool skin may occasionally be secondary to hypothyroidism. Other cutaneous findings include alopecia of the lateral eyebrows, non-pitting edema and a diffuse, non-scarring alopecia.

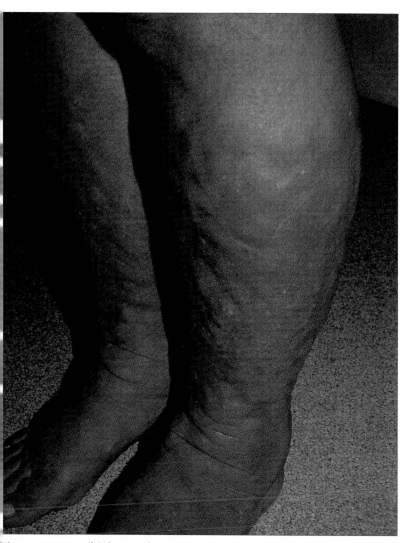

Figure 545. Pretibial myxedema. Skin-colored or red–brown plaques of the pretibial area of a hyperthyroid patient are characteristic. Various clinical forms have been described, including non-pitting edema (most common), the plaque form, the nodular form and the elephantiasic form (as shown here). Almost all patients have high levels of thyroid stimulating antibodies. The vast majority of patients also have ophthalmopathy which may be severe, to the point of requiring decompressive surgery.

283

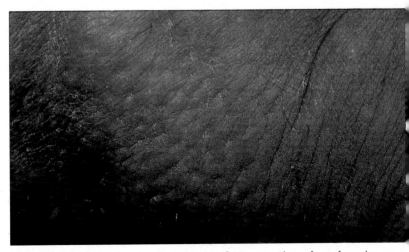

Figure 546. Pretibial myxedema, peau d'orange. The surface often takes on the appearance of an orange, so-called peau d'orange.

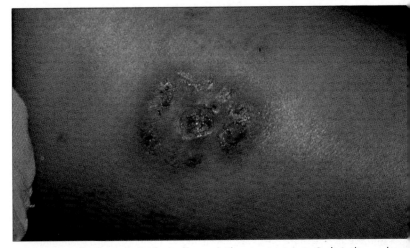

Figure 547. Metastatic Crohn's disease. The term metastatic Crohn's disease has been used to describe cutaneous granuloma formation in a patient with Crohn's disease.

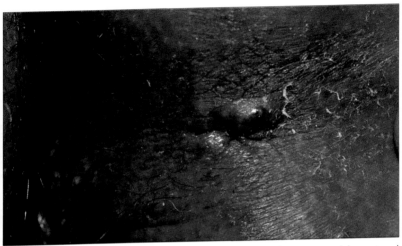

Figure 548. Anal fistula. A fistulous connection between the rectum and the perianal skin may occur. Flatus may emanate, confirming the diagnosis.

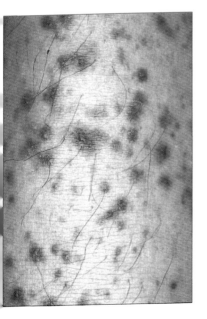

Figure 549. Scurvy. Perifollicular hemorrhage, corkscrew hairs on the legs, easy bleeding and hypertrophy of the gums, purpura and epistaxis all occur in scurvy, a deficiency of vitamin C. Patients whose diets may be deficient enough to develop scurvy include elderly, poor, mentally ill or alcoholic individuals. (Courtesy of Eliot Mostow, MD.)

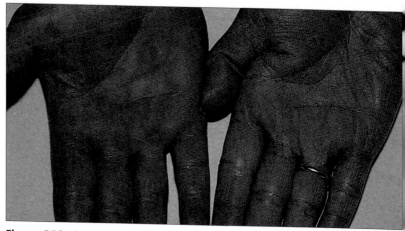

Figure 550. Carotenemia. A diffuse orangish discoloration of the palms in a patient who eats large quantities of carrots occurs in carotenemia. In contrast to jaundice, the eyes are not icteric.

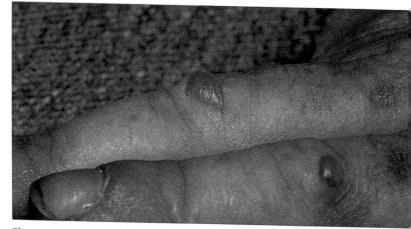

Figure 551. Porphyria cutanea tarda. Vesicles, milia, erosions and fragile skin occur symmetrically on the dorsa of the hands in porphyria cutanea tarda. Both an autosomal dominant inherited and an acquired type have been described. For both types, uroporphyrinogen decarboxylase functional activity is low and a history of exposure to alcohol, estrogens or a liver toxic agent may be found. Hepatitis C virus infection may be found in acquired porphyria cutanea tarda.

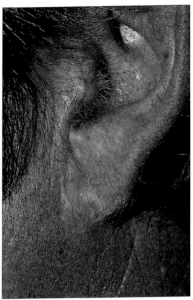

Figure 552. Porphyria cutanea tarda, hypertrichosis. Look for hypertrichosis along the forehead and on the ears, as shown here.

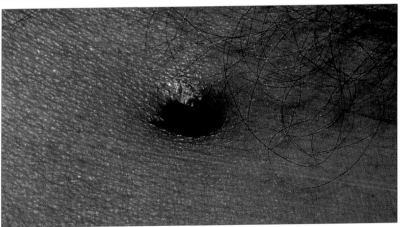

Figure 553. Metastatic lung cancer. Unexplained skin nodules, non-healing ulcers or persistent indurated erythema may all be manifestations of cutaneous metastatic disease. The principal sites for cutaneous metastasis are the scalp, chest and abdomen. These lesions may represent a direct extension or hematogenous spread. The most common solid tumors to metastasize to the skin are cancers of the breast and colon and melanoma.

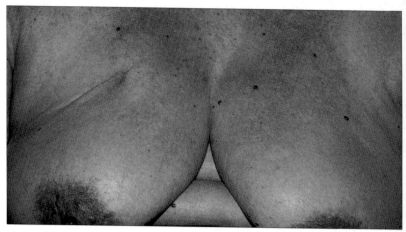

Figure 554. Breast cancer. Nipple or skin retraction or breast asymmetry may develop with breast cancer. A subcutaneous nodule or induration may occur. Skin retraction is seen on the upper part of this woman's breast.

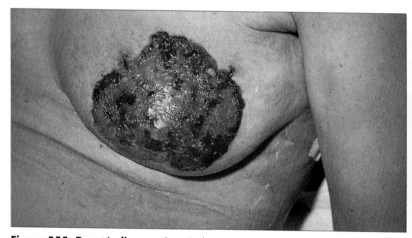

Figure 555. Paget's disease. Paget's disease represents cutaneous invasion by an underlying ductal carcinoma. A chronic, slowly enlarging, sharply demarcated, red, scaly lesion of the nipple and/or breast occurs. There may be ulceration, infiltration or an underlying, palpable mass. Often, however, the mammogram is normal and no palpable mass is found. The condition is typically mistaken for eczema and treated with topical steroids for years. (Courtesy of Gary Cole, MD.)

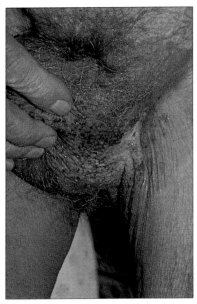

Figure 556. Extramammary Paget's disease. Extramammary Paget's disease presents in an older adult as a slowly expanding exudative, eczematous or red plaque in the groin, perianal area or axilla. Each lesion falls into one of three categories: i) unassociated with an underlying malignancy, presumably representing *in situ* malignant transformation of the intraepidermal component of the sweat duct, ii) epidermotropic spread from an adjacent apocrine or eccrine gland carcinoma or iii) epidermotropic spread or metastasis from an underlying cancer (e.g. bladder, rectum, urethra, cervix or breast).

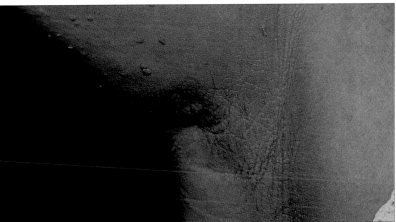

Figure 557. Acanthosis nigricans, malignant. The onset of a severe acanthosis nigricans in an adult without diabetes or obesity may suggest an occult malignancy, often of gastric origin. This patient complained of recent thickening of the skin of the axilla and neck as well as the development of multiple tags. An esophageal cancer was found. (See also **Figure 536**.)

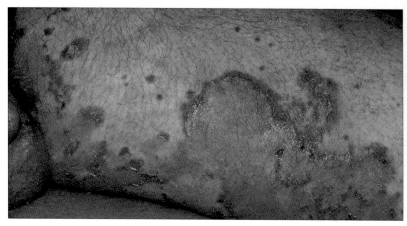

Figure 558. Necrolytic migratory erythema. An annular, erosive or bullous eruption develops periorally and in the groin in necrolytic migratory erythema. Weight loss, anemia, diabetes mellitus and glossitis may occur. A glucagon-secreting, alpha cell tumor of the pancreas is the usual cause, although some patients may have necrolytic migratory erythema without a glucagonoma.

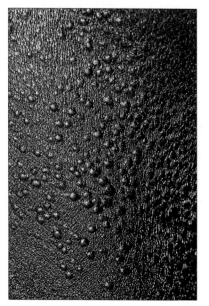

Figure 559. Lichen myxedematosis. Diffuse deposition of mucin in the skin is the cause of this disease, and innumerable uniform 2–3 mm skin-colored papules along the arms, neck and face result. When confluent with underlying induration, the term scleromyxedema is used. An associated paraprotein is usually found and is most commonly of the IgG-lambda type. Mucin deposition may occur internally, although life expectancy is usually not affected.

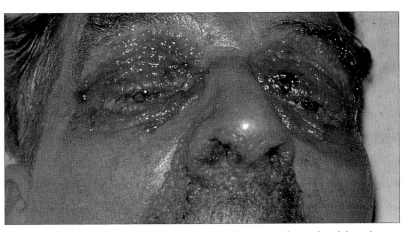

Figure 560. Systemic amyloidosis. Periorbital waxy papules and nodules, along with petechiae and purpura after the slightest trauma (pinch purpura) are characteristic of this infiltrative disease. Post-proctoscopic periorbital purpura is a classic but uncommon presentation. A paraprotein is found in the majority, and approximately one-third of patients have an associated myeloma. (Courtesy of Department of Dermatology, UCSD.)

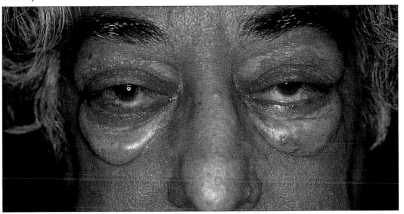

Figure 561. Necrobiotic xanthogranuloma with paraproteinemia.
Periorbital yellow nodules and plaques that may ulcerate occur in necrobiotic xanthogranuloma. Lesions may be violaceous or xanthomatous and may occur anywhere on the extremities or trunk. Serum protein electrophoresis shows a paraprotein. Keratitis, scleritis and anterior uveitis may occur as well as hepatosplenomegaly. Bone marrow plasmacytosis is common but multiple myeloma is rare. (Courtesy of Theodore Sebastian, MD.)

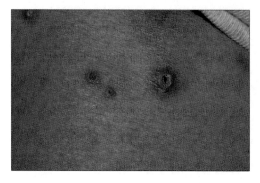

Figure 562. Perforating disorder of dialysis.
Hyperkeratotic papules on the thighs of a patient with renal failure (usually from diabetes mellitus) and on dialysis are characteristic. Material from the dermis is being extruded through the central hyperkeratotic core of each papule. Lesions may be very pruritic and a component of prurigo nodularis may be present.

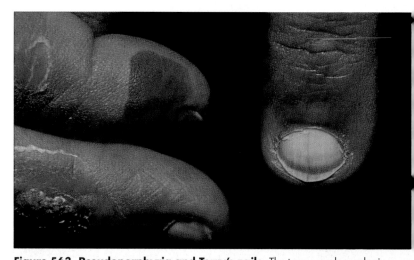

Figure 563. Pseudoporphyria and Terry's nails. The term pseudoporphyria refers to vesicles and fragility on the dorsa of the hands resulting from exposure to both a weak sensitizer (e.g. a sulfonamide, dapsone, furosemide, nalidixic acid, naproxen, pyridoxone, fluoroquinolone antibiotics or tetracycline) and significant ultraviolet light (e.g. from the sun or a tanning bed). The clinical presentation is nearly identical to porphyria cutanea tarda (thus pseudoporphyria). However, urine porphyrin levels are normal and hypertrichosis is absent. Patients with renal failure, and especially those on dialysis, are at increased risk for developing this condition. Terry's nails are also present in this patient (white nail with distal pink rim).

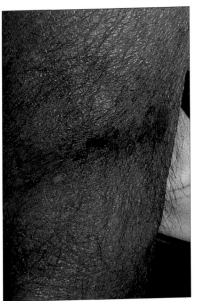

Figure 564. Calciphylaxis. Painful mottling of the skin resembling livedo reticularis in a patient with chronic renal failure on dialysis is characteristic of the initial lesion. Later, these areas become indurated, echymotic plaques that enlarge and develop central necrosis and ulceration. Distal gangrene and autoamputation of multiple digits are common. Extensive calcification of blood vessels may be seen histologically and on X-rays.

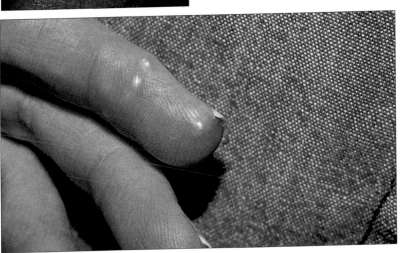

Figure 565. Gout. Yellowish-white papules on the fingertips may rarely occur as a manifestation of gout. Whitish or flesh-colored papulonodules may also occur on the rim of the ears, elbows and over the knuckles. These tophi are deposits of monosodium urate crystals. Special fixation of the skin biopsy is needed so as not to dissolve the urate crystals.

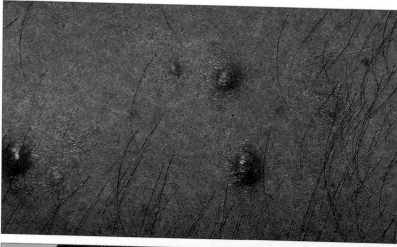

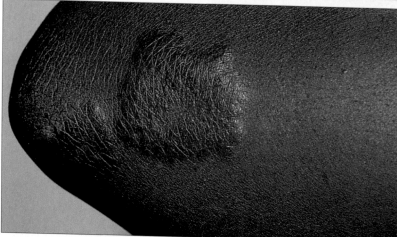

Figures 566 and 567. Sarcoidosis. Sarcoidosis may manifest itself in the skin in many ways including papules (**Figure 566**), plaques (**Figure 567**), nodules, annular lesions, ulcers, ichthyosis, scar infiltration, erythroderma, lupus pernio (**Figure 568**), ungual lesions, hypopigmented plaques (**Figure 569**) and erythema nodosum. Ocular (uveitis, iris nodules, conjunctivitis), pulmonary, musculoskelatal (polyarthritis, bone cysts) and lymph node involvement are common. Granulomas may be found in the kidneys, heart and elsewhere.

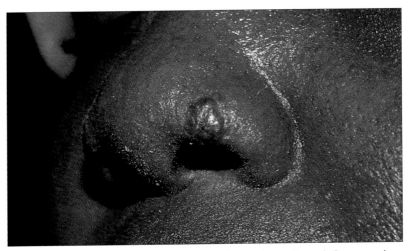

Figure 568. Sarcoidosis, lupus pernio. Red, smooth papules and plaques on the nose and other acral areas, such as the ears, fingers and toes, occur in lupus pernio, a subtype of sarcoidosis. Bone cysts of the fingers may be associated.

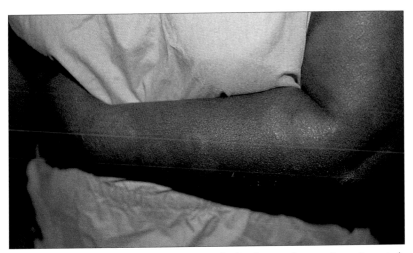

Figure 569. Sarcoidosis, hypopigmented. The skin may become hypopigmented over plaques of sarcoidosis.

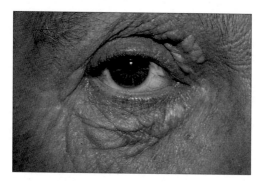

Figure 570.
Xanthelasma. Soft, yellow plaques on the upper, inner eyelids are characteristic of xanthelasma. They may occur as an isolated finding or in association with a hyperlipidemia.

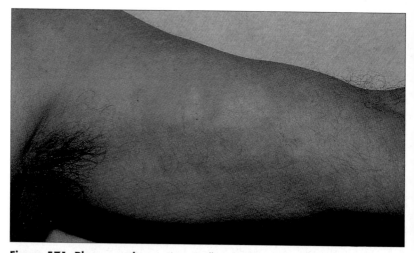

Figure 571. Plane xanthoma. Large yellow patches or very slightly elevated yellow plaques are characteristic and are illustrated here on the arm of this patient with myeloma. Plane xanthomas may be subdivided into 3 groups: i) associated with other xanthomas and part of a familial hyperlipidemia or secondary to liver disease, usually biliary cirrhosis, ii) associated with a paraprotein and elevated lipids, iii) associated with a paraprotein but no elevation in the lipids. In groups ii and iii, the paraprotein seems to interfere with lipid metabolism and may cause a lipoprotein–paraprotein complex with either elevation of the lipids or increase in their phagocytosis by macrophages.

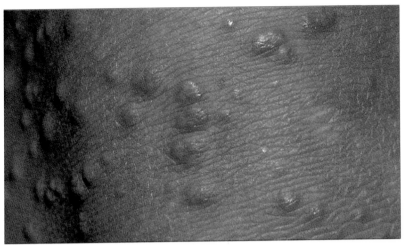

Figure 572. Eruptive xanthoma. A widespread, symmetric eruption of yellow papules with preference for the knees, elbows and buttocks occurs in eruptive xanthoma. Conditions that predispose to the eruption include diabetes mellitus, chronic renal failure, nephrotic syndrome, hypothyroidism, alcohol ingestion, underlying hypertriglyceridemia and certain drugs (e.g. isotretinoin).

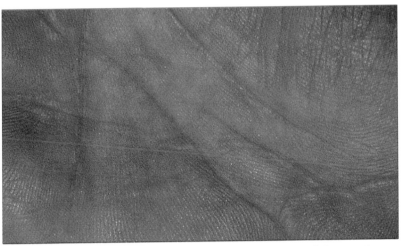

Figure 573. Xanthoma palmare. Xanthoma palmare is a type of plane xanthoma and presents as yellow palmar creases. It usually occurs in type III (broad beta) hyperlipidemia. (Courtesy of Stephen H Ducatman, MD.)

Sun Damage/
Non-Melanoma Skin Cancers

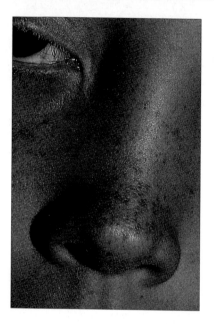

Figure 574. Freckles/ephelides.
Light tan or brown macules scattered on the face or nose of a light-skinned, red-haired patient are characteristic. The nose is preferentially affected as it receives sunlight more directly. The health-care provider should encourage the parents of affected children to put on the sunscreen.

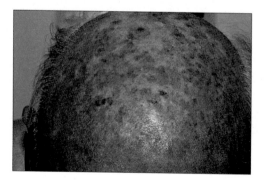

Figure 575.
Photodamaged skin, scalp. Aged skin without sun damage is thin and lacking in subcutaneous fat. Chronic photodamage adds mottled pigmentation, solar elastosis, additional wrinkling and, to the susceptible, actinic keratoses, basal cell and squamous cell carcinomas. Hats are an essential part of protection, especially as the hair thins.

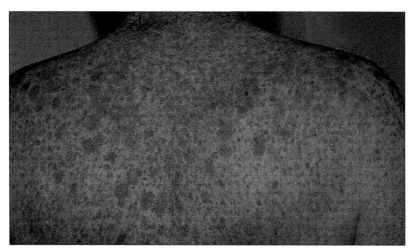

Figure 576. Mottled pigmentation. Chronic sun exposure may lead to multiple brown macules or lentigines. Hypopigmentation and telangiectasias may also develop. Melanomas of course may also occur and so all pigmented lesions should be evaluated by the ABCD criteria (see **Figure 452**) and if two are present, a biopsy should be performed.

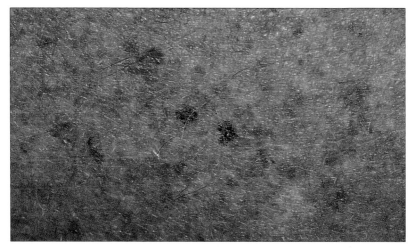

Figure 577. Lentigo, ink dot. An especially dark, irregularly pigmented macule like an ink drop may occur on the upper back and is completely benign.

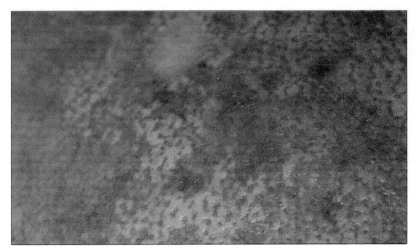

Figure 578. Solar elastosis. A reticulate pattern of yellow papules is seen below the thinned skin. The forehead of men with a receding hairline is most commonly affected.

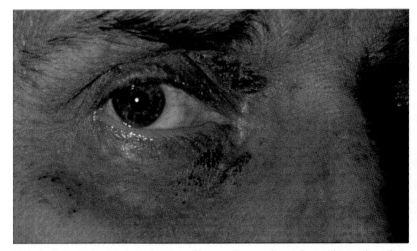

Figure 579. Favre–Racouchot syndrome. Cysts, milia and comedones about the lateral eyes and cheeks in a middle-aged to elderly patient with a significant history of sun exposure are characteristic. Note the tremendous number of comedones about the eyes in this patient.

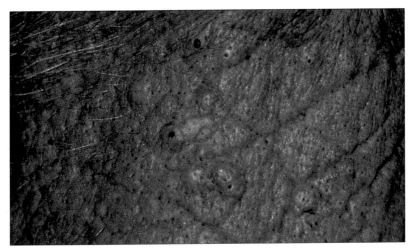

Figure 580. Cutis rhomboidalis nuchae/Favre–Racouchot syndrome.
Diagonal furrows that criss-cross the nape forming rhomboids in an older patient after much sun exposure are characteristic of cutis rhomboidalis nuchae. Cysts and comedones of Favre–Racouchot syndrome are also seen.

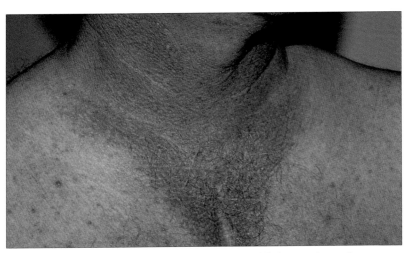

Figure 581. Poikiloderma of Civatte. The term poikiloderma refers to the combination of mottled pigmentation, telangiectasias and cutaneous atrophy. It may occur about the neck as a result of chronic sun exposure.

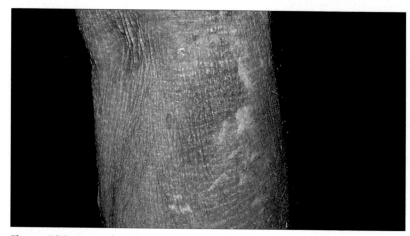

Figure 582. Age-related purpura. Red–purple patches 1–4 cm in size on the exterior forearms or dorsa of the hands in the older photodamaged arm are characteristic of age-related purpura. These bruises are precipitated by the slightest trauma. Old age and chronic steroid use, especially intramuscularly, predisposes to these lesions. Other terms that have been used include senile purpura and solar purpura.

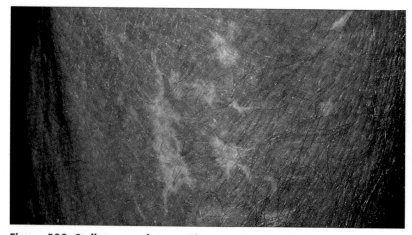

Figure 583. Stellate pseudoscars. These irregular, white, linear or star-shaped lesions occur on the sun-exposed forearms of older people. Chronic steroid use may predispose the patient to their formation.

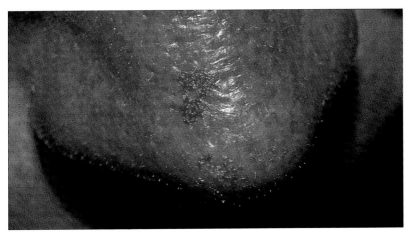

Figure 584. Actinic keratosis, nose. A fixed, hyperkeratotic or scaly papule on the face, arms or hands of an adult is characteristic of this premalignant, UV-induced condition. The patient often complains of a burning or itching sensation. The scaly papule periodically falls off—often just before the doctor's appointment! These lesions are often better felt than seen, and thus the doctor should not be afraid to touch the patient in order to find them.

Figure 585. Actinic keratosis, face, multiple. Multiple actinic keratoses are seen on this man's left cheek and temple. The presence of multiple actinic keratoses is one of the strongest predictors of future basal cell carcinoma (BCC) and squamous cell carcinoma (SCC). Regular sunscreen use, sun avoidance and a low fat diet reduce their numbers.

303

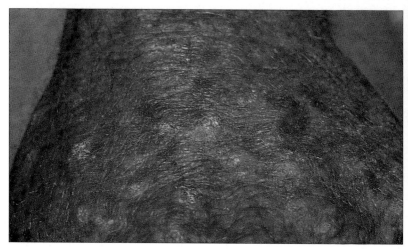

Figure 586. Actinic keratoses, dorsa hand. Older individuals with a history of chronic sun exposure may develop hyperkeratotic papules or scaly areas on the dorsa of the hands. The majority represent hypertrophic actinic keratoses (as shown here). The differential diagnosis for large lesions would include a SCC and, if rapidly growing, a keratoacanthoma. Basal cell carcinoma for some reason is rare on the dorsa of the hands.

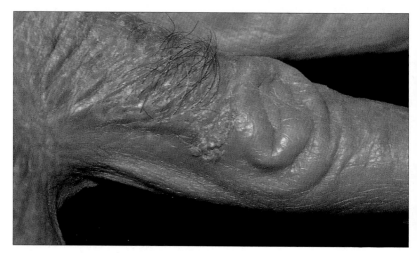

Figure 587. Actinic keratosis, finger. The dorsa of the fingers should not be forgotten during a cutaneous examination.

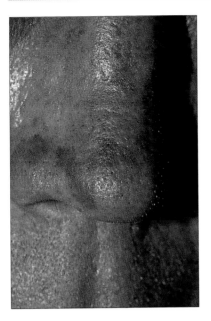

Figure 588. Actinic keratosis, spreading pigmented. A slowly expanding brown patch or plaque on the face of a chronically sun-damaged adult is characteristic. The surface of this lesion is usually scaly, rough or hyperkeratotic in comparison to a solar lentigo.

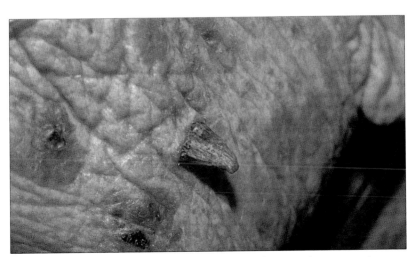

Figure 589. Actinic keratosis, cutaneous horn. This conical projection of compact hyperkeratosis usually overlies an actinic keratosis, although a SCC, seborrheic keratosis or verruca may be found.

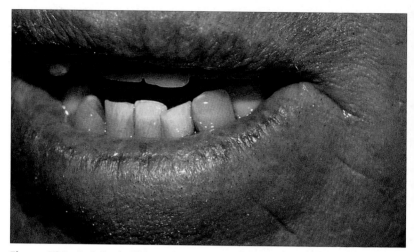

Figure 590. Actinic cheilitis. A fixed hyperkeratotic papule or diffuse scale on the lower lip is characteristic of actinic cheilitis, which is a common premalignant condition occurring after years of sun exposure. Palpation for induration or thickening that might signal an underlying squamous cell carcinoma is critically important.

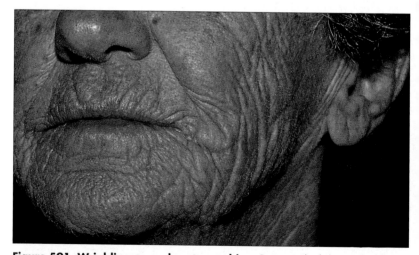

Figure 591. Wrinkling secondary to smoking. Patients who have smoked for more than 50 pack-years are almost 5 times as likely to be wrinkled as non-smokers. Deep furrows on the cheeks and jaw and wrinkles radiating out from the lips and eyes are characteristic of wrinkles related to smoking.

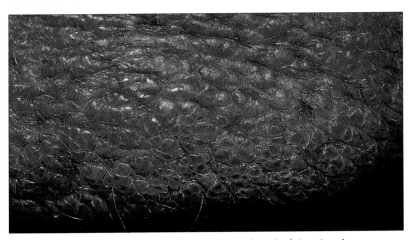

Figure 592. Colloid milia. This condition is the end result of decades of sun exposure. Firm papules on the dorsa of the hands, arms (as shown here), forehead or cheeks in an older patient are characteristic.

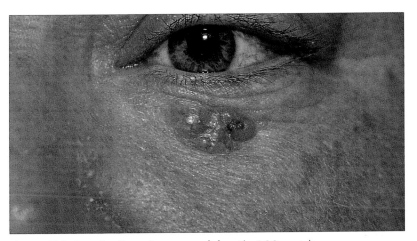

Figure 593. Basal cell carcinoma, nodular. The BCC can take on many appearances. A slowly expanding pearly papule with telangiectasias on the face of an older person is classic. Risk factors for facial skin cancer include sunbed use, radio-therapy, a family history of skin cancers, type I skin, a tendency to freckle in childhood and Irish, Scottish, Scandinavian or German heritage. Routine follow-up should occur for any patient with BCC as approximately 40% will develop a second BCC within 5 years.

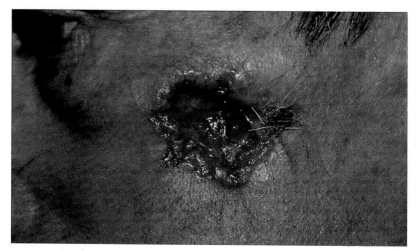

Figure 594. Basal cell carcinoma, rodent ulcer. If untreated, the nodule expands and undergoes central ulceration. The edge is often described as having a rolled border. The term rodent ulcer is sometimes used, as if a rat had gnawed a hole in the skin.

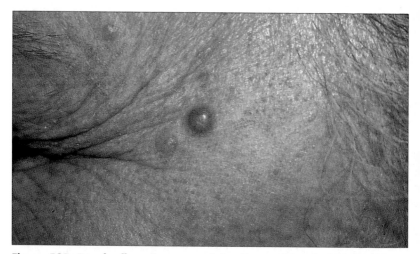

Figure 595. Basal cell carcinoma, nodular. The possibility of a BCC should be considered with any slowly growing papule or nodule on the face of a fair-skinned adult. It may be clinically impossible to distinguish a flesh-colored nevus from a BCC. The reddish papule with telangiectasias in the center of the photograph is a BCC. The smaller papule to the left and below is a benign nevus.

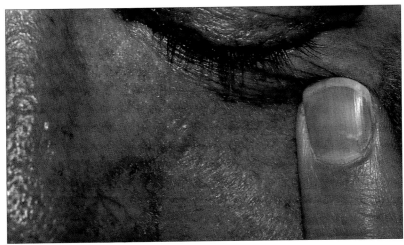

Figure 596. Basal cell carcinoma, morpheaform. The morpheaform or fibrosing BCC often has a whitish or yellowish hue. It is typically flat or even depressed and the margins ill-defined.

Figure 597. Superficial basal cell carcinoma. This variant of BCC usually presents as a slowly enlarging, red, scaly area on the back of an older adult with significant sun exposure. Ulceration is unusual. The process is limited to the superficial layers of the skin.

Figure 598. Basal cell carcinoma, recurrent. The follow-up examination of any patient with a history of a BCC should include an examination with palpation of the scar for recurrence. Surface changes including redness, scale or crust should arouse suspicion, as well as a new dermal papule. In the figure, redness and slight scale just superior to the whitish scar represents a recurrence of a superficial BCC which had previously undergone electrodesiccation and curettage.

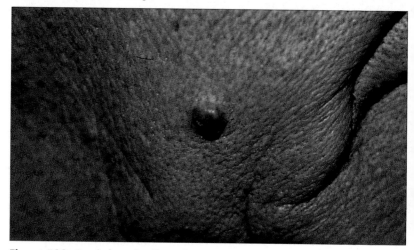

Figure 599. Cystic basal cell carcinoma. A blue–purple, dermal nodule is typical of this uncommon variant of BCC. The cyst is formed by necrosis and degeneration of the center of a solid (nodular) BCC.

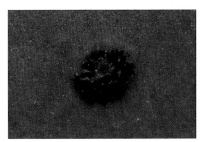

Figure 600. Pigmented basal cell in a Filipino man. This variant is similar to the nodular BCC except for the abundant pigment. Such lesions may mimic melanoma. Dark-skinned but not Black patients are at greatest risk. (See also **Figure 449**.)

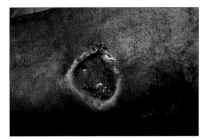

Figure 601. Basal cell carcinoma mimicking chronic stasis ulcer. Occasionally, an ulcer on the leg may represent a BCC or an SCC. Often, such lesions are treated for years as a stasis ulcer. (Photograph courtesy of Michael O Murphy, MD.)

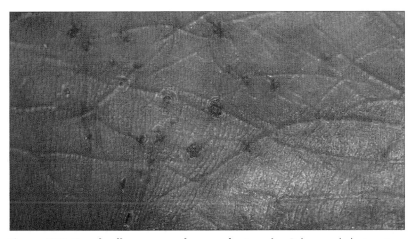

Figure 602. Basal cell nevus syndrome, plantar pits. Palmar and plantar pits and a tendency towards multiple BCCs of the face and trunk occur in this autosomal dominant syndrome. Associated abnormalities involve the CNS (e.g. mental retardation, calcification of the falx cerebri, congenital hydrocephalus-macrocephaly, meduloblastoma, meningioma, cysts), bones (e.g. a characteristic fascies, a marfanoid habitus, fused, bifid or missing ribs, odontogenic keratocysts of the jaw, vertebral abnormalities) and eyes (e.g. congenital cataracts, glaucoma).

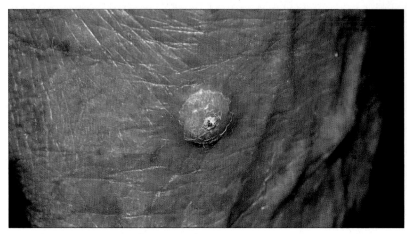

Figure 603. Keratoacanthoma, early. A rapidly growing nodule that develops a central keratotic core in the sun-exposed area of an elderly person is characteristic. The hands and arms as well as the head and neck are commonly affected. The distinction between keratoacanthoma and SCC may be blurred histologically, as was true in this case. Chronic UV exposure seems to be a predisposing factor and the patient should be examined for other non-melanoma skin cancers.

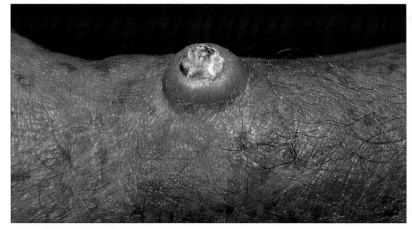

Figure 604. Keratoacanthoma. This figure shows the classic features of a mature lesion. A dome-shaped nodule with a central horn-filled core is seen. Growth to this size usually takes about 2 months.

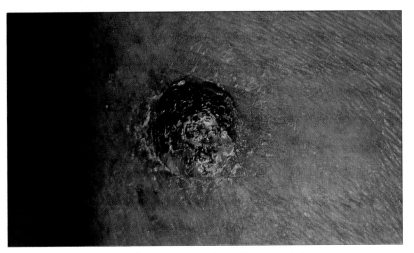

Figure 605. Keratoacanthoma, regressing. If left untreated, most keratoacanthomas regress, usually within 6 months.

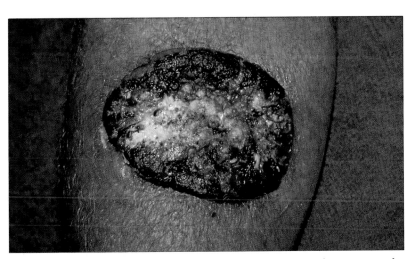

Figure 606. Keratoacanthoma, giant. Although most keratoacanthomas regress if left untreated, a small percentage do not. A progressively enlarging verrucous lesion with central clearing or atrophy is the result. The periphery of the lesion shows typical features of keratoacanthoma whereas the center may show atrophy and dermal scarring. Diameters of 5–30 cm have been reported.

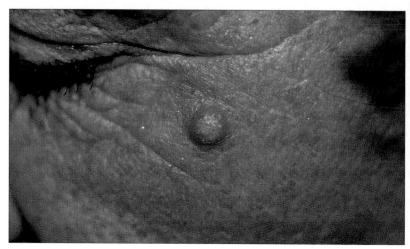

Figure 607. Squamous cell carcinoma, small. A hyperkeratotic, enlarging plaque or nodule usually in a photoexposed area of an older adult is characteristic. Those on the lip, within scars and in areas not exposed to the sun must be considered more aggressive but even small SCCs in sun-exposed areas may metastasize. Those patients at increased risk for SCC have light skin, blonde or red hair, a tendency to burn rather than tan in the sun and chronic occupational solar exposure.

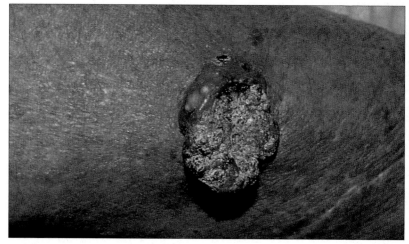

Figure 608. Squamous cell carcinoma, large.

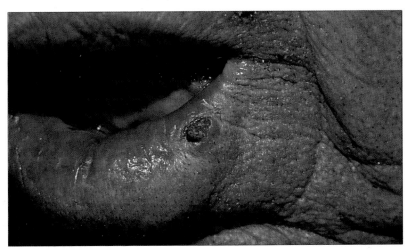

Figure 609. Squamous cell carcinoma, lip. Actinic cheilitis (**Figure 590**) may progress to invasive SCC. A slowly enlarging, hyperkeratotic papulonodule originating from the vermilion border of the lower lip is characteristic. Squamous cell carcinoma of the lip has a higher incidence of metastasis compared with cutaneous SCC.

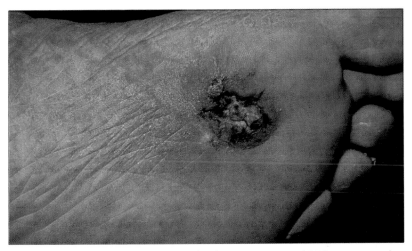

Figure 610. Verrucous carcinoma. This slow-growing type of SCC common on the sole resembles a wart. Indeed, some of these lesions may have begun as a wart. (Photograph courtesy of Gary Cole, MD.)

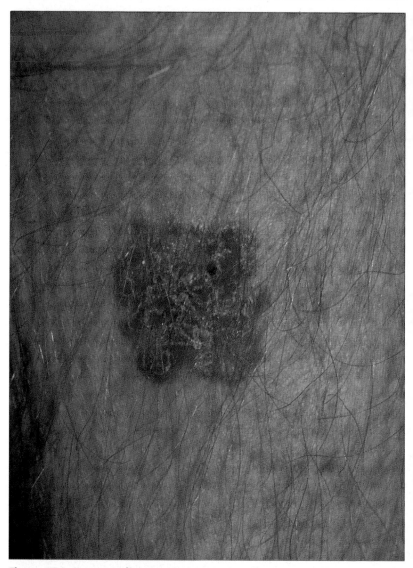

Figure 611. Bowen's disease. The term Bowen's disease is used for SCC *in situ* that has a characteristic histopathologic picture. Clinically, one finds a slowly enlarging, sharply demarcated, red, scaly plaque. It may occur on sun-exposed or sun-protected sites. Many patients have a history of either BCC or SCC.

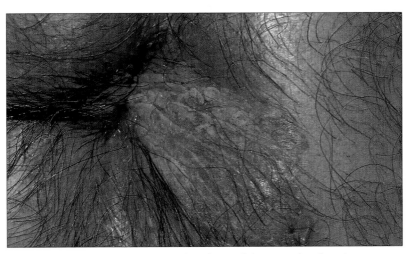

Figure 612. Bowen's disease, perianal. A well-demarcated, red, scaly, moist plaque in the perianal area that is slow growing over years is characteristic.

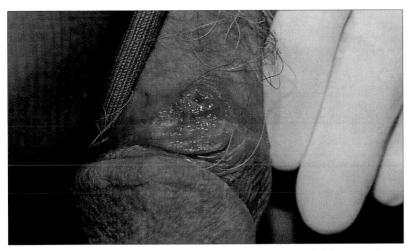

Figure 613. Erythroplasia of Queyrat. A fixed red, moist patch/plaque on the glans of an uncircumcised elderly man is characteristic of this disease, which represents SCC *in situ*. An underlying invasive SCC may be found.

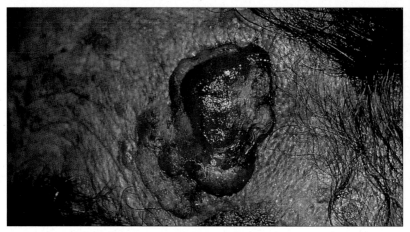

Figure 614. Atypical fibroxanthoma, ulcerative nodule. A solitary papule that grows to an ulcerated nodule on the head or neck in an older White person is characteristic. Bleeding and ulceration are common. Metastasis may rarely occur. Immunohistochemical studies are needed to exclude SCC and melanoma.

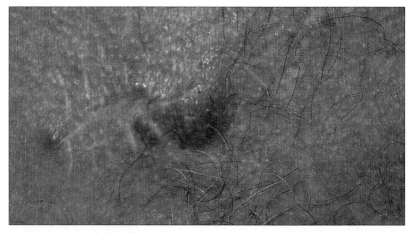

Figure 615. Merkel cell. A solitary, red–purple or violaceous, shiny, dome-shaped nodule or plaque on the face, head or neck of an elderly person is characteristic. Twenty percent occur in the periorbital area. Local recurrence and spread to regional lymph nodes and distant sites are characteristic with significant mortality. (Courtesy of Duane Whitaker, MD.)

Tumors and Nodules

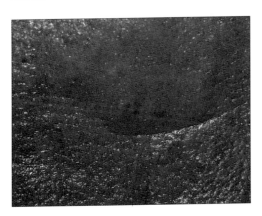

Figure 616. Sebaceous hyperplasia. These 2–4 mm 'yellow donuts' develop on the face with age. Favored sites are the forehead, temples and cheeks. There is no correlation with sun exposure or solar elastosis.

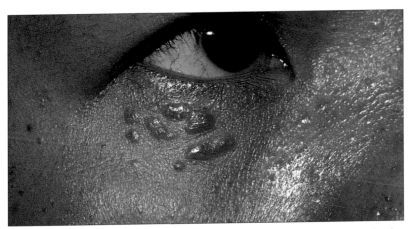

Figure 617. Syringomas, periorbital. These tumorous collections of sweat glands commonly occur infra-orbitally in patients of Asian descent. Rarely, they may be distributed diffusely on the face or body or be present as a solitary lesion.

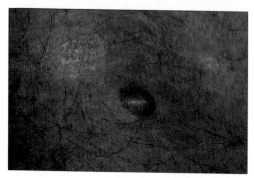

Figure 618. Neuro-fibroma. A soft, flesh-colored, non-descript papule is characteristic. One may be able to buttonhole the lesion through the skin. Multiple neurofibromas occur in neurofibromatosis (see **Figure 56**).

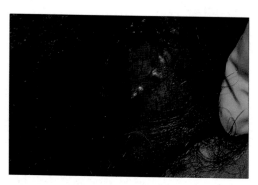

Figure 619. Hidradenoma papilliferum. A solitary dermal papule or nodule in the vulvar or perivulvar area is characteristic of this adnexal tumor of apocrine origin.

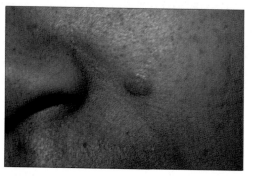

Figure 620. Tricho-epithelioma, solitary. This papule, usually located on the face, commonly resembles a nevus or a basal cell carcinoma. A yellowish-white color and a depressed center are distinguishing features.

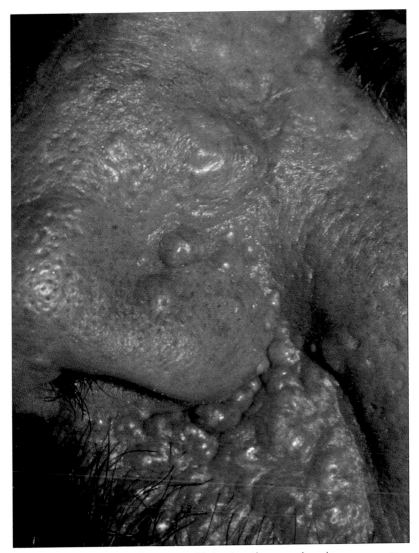

Figure 621. Trichoepithelioma, multiple. As with many adnexal tumors, trichoepitheliomas may occur multiply inherited as an autosomal dominant trait. Multiple, symmetric, flesh-colored papules occur characteristically along the nasolabial folds and upper lip, with onset in the teens. Lesions on the ear and forehead also occur. Cylindromas of the scalp may be associated.

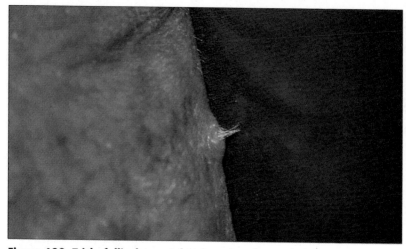

Figure 622. Trichofolliculoma. A facial papule with several white, wispy hairs emanating from the center is characteristic.

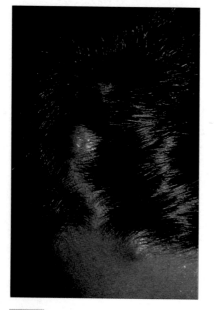

Figure 623. Cylindroma.
Cylindromas present as solitary or multiple, firm, dermal nodules on the scalp. When multiple, the condition is often inherited autosomal dominantly and trichoepitheliomas may be associated. (Courtesy of Michael O Murphy, MD.)

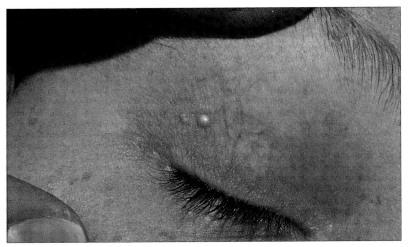

Figure 624. Milia. A woman will commonly complain about these tiny, facial 'white heads' that just will not 'pop'. In reality, they represent miniature epidermal inclusion cysts.

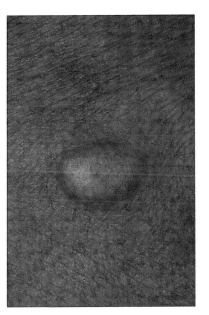

Figure 625. Epidermal inclusion cyst. A dermal nodule, at times with a visible pore, is a common occurrence in adults. Lesions typically occur on the back, neck and face. When superficial, the nodule may be whitish in color. The lesion grows slowly over time and may periodically drain. The patient commonly complains that the extruded material is foul smelling.

323

Figure 626. Epidermal inclusion cyst, ruptured. Occasionally, the cyst wall of an epidermal inclusion cyst ruptures into the dermis causing an intense inflammatory foreign body response. Swelling, erythema and pain occur. The inflammation may remain deep and slowly resolve over weeks to a month or it may become fluctuant and drain spontaneously, as shown here.

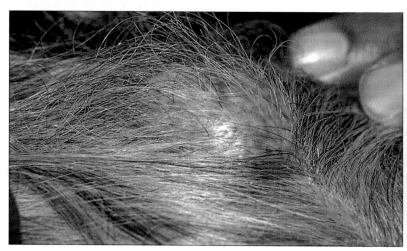

Figure 627. Pilar cyst. This type of cyst occurs almost exclusively on the scalp. It is firm, round and usually non-tender. When multiple, it may be inherited autosomal dominantly.

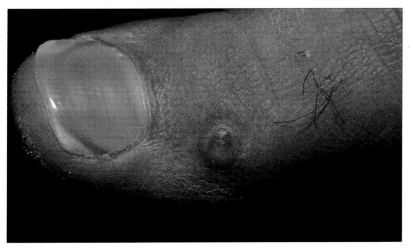

Figure 628. Digital mucous cyst. This pseudocyst contains a clear, viscous fluid representing an abnormal production of ground substance. Why it prefers the area between the distal interphalangeal joint and the nail is unknown. If it impinges on the nail matrix, a groove may form in the nail plate (see **Figure 420**). Hemorrhage into the lesions may occur, turning them blue or black.

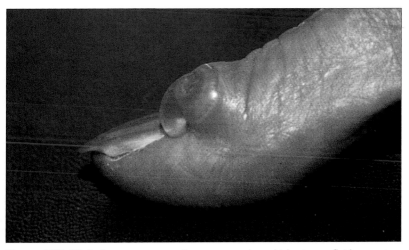

Figure 629. Digital mucous cyst. On rupture, a clear, thick, viscous fluid emanates.

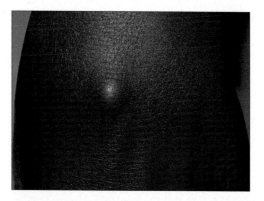

Figure 630. Ganglion cyst. A 1–3 cm subcutaneous nodule overlying the ankle or wrist may represent a ganglion cyst.

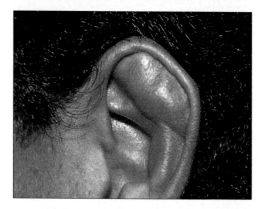

Figure 631. Pseudocyst, ear. A non-tender, firm, cystic lesion of the ear is characteristic. It may be preceded by trauma as occurred in two boys after ear pulling for their birthday. It also may be associated with atopic dermatitis. Drainage yields a thick, viscous fluid.

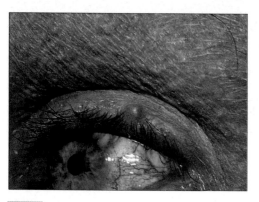

Figure 632. Apocrine hydrocystoma. A solitary, flesh-colored to bluish, cystic lesion about the eyes is characteristic.

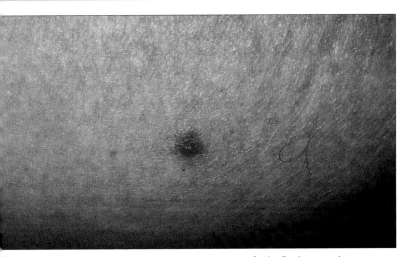

Figure 633. Apocrine hydrocystoma, pigmented. The fluid secreted into an apocrine hydrocystoma may be so dark blue–black that the lesion may appear nevomelanocytic.

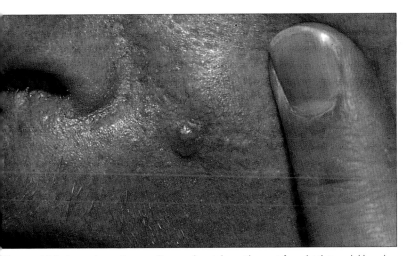

Figure 634. Lymphangioma. Grouped vesicles with onset from birth to adulthood are characteristic of lymphangioma circumscriptum. Their appearance has been likened to frog spawn. The fluid may be blood-tinged or show a blood/fluid line. These lesions often communicate with deeper lymphatics.

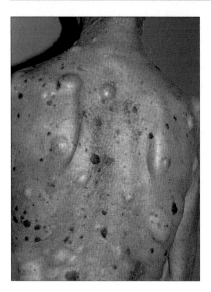

Figure 635. Steatocystoma multiplex. Multiple, soft, cystic papulonodules develop on the chest, back, axilla and elsewhere in steatocystoma multiplex. They may range from 2 mm to 4 cm in size. The contents ranges from milky-white to clear and oily. Rupture, inflammation and scarring of individual cysts may occur. Inheritance is autosomal dominant.

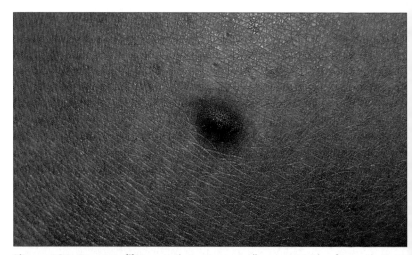

Figure 636. Dermatofibroma. The patient typically presents with a firm, red, brown or flesh-colored papule on the leg. The surface may be smooth, hyperkeratotic or velvety. The upper back and arms are other possibly sites. Multiple dermatofibromas (e.g. more than 15) have been associated with various diseases including lupus erythematosus.

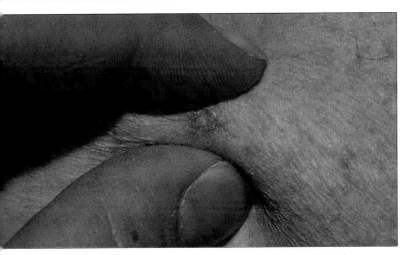

Figure 637. Dermatofibroma, buttonhole sign. Application of lateral pressure causes the center to dimple.

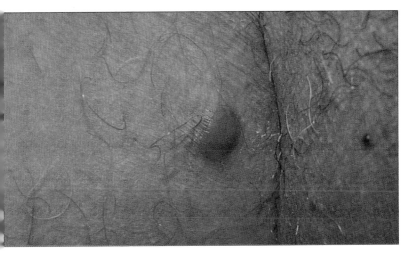

Figure 638. Fibrohistiocytoma. This benign neoplasm is akin to the dermatofibroma but histologically is more cellular with less epidermal change. The patient usually presents with one or more flesh-colored to pink–red firm dermal nodules.

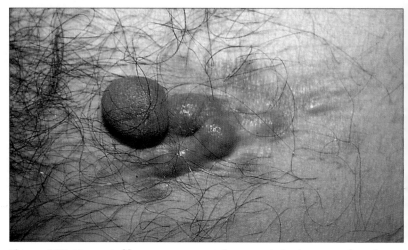

Figure 639. Dermatofibrosarcoma protuberans. A slowly growing firm plaque that later becomes multinodular on the trunk or proximal extremities in an adult is characteristic. Congenital lesions have been reported and lesions have occurred at sites of a previous trauma e.g. vaccination site, bayonet wound. Metastases are rare with this malignant tumor but local recurrence after surgery is common. (Courtesy of Michael O Murphy, MD.)

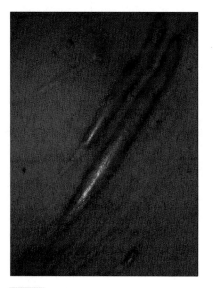

Figure 640. Hypertrophic scar. An elevated and excessive growth of fibrous tissue within and not extending beyond the bounds of a scar is characteristic. Hypertrophic scars usually resolve over time, whereas keloids usually do not. This patient's hypertrophic scars developed after a motorcycle accident.

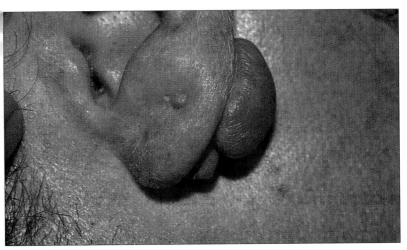

Figure 641. Keloid, earlobe. A firm, rubbery nodule on the lobe usually on the posterior surface after ear piercing is characteristic. Young people and Blacks are most commonly affected by keloids. Other favored sites include the neck, shoulders and back. Note the two keloids after two ear piercings.

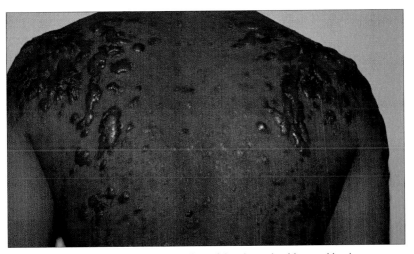

Figure 642. Keloid, diffuse. The midline of the chest, shoulders and back are favorite locations for the formation of firm, rubbery papular or nodular keloids.

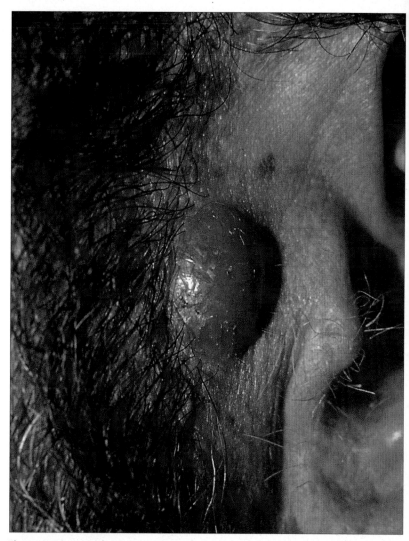

Figure 643. Lymphocytoma cutis. This nodule represents a dermal collection of inflammatory cells with an abundance of lymphocytes. Clinically, a 0.5–2 cm asymptomatic, erythematous to plum-colored papule or nodule is seen. They may occur virtually anywhere with a special predilection for the face and ears. A skin biopsy, complete blood count and lymph node examination are reasonable to help exclude malignancy.

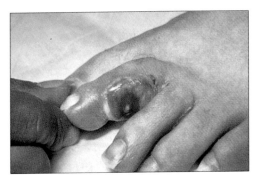

Figure 644. Lymphoma cutis. A lymphoma may rarely present in the skin. Clinically, one sees solitary or multiple, red papulonodules. The clinical differentiation between lymphoma and pseudo-lymphoma may be difficult. (Courtesy of Michael O Murphy, MD.)

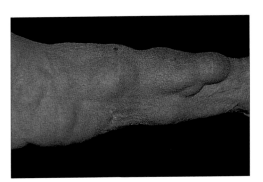

Figure 645. Lipoma, multiple. A lipoma represents a subcutaneous collection of fat. It may be solitary or multiple. The back is a favored site. Unlike an epidermal inclusion cyst, the lipoma has no pore and the overlying skin is movable and unattached to the lesion.

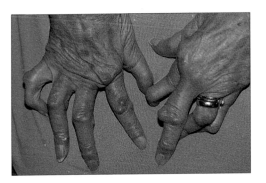

Figure 646. Rheumatoid nodule. Patients with rheumatoid arthritis may develop these nodules over bony prominences such as the knuckles and elbows. These nodules most commonly occur in association with rheumatoid arthritis but may also be seen in systemic lupus erythema-tosus and scleroderma.

Urticarias

Figure 647. Urticaria.
Itchy, edematous, raised, pink plaques without scale that move and change daily are characteristic. Annular lesions resulting from central clearing and white halos (like the Woronoff's ring of psoriasis) can occur. Delayed pressure urticaria, angioedema and dermatographism may accompany urticaria.

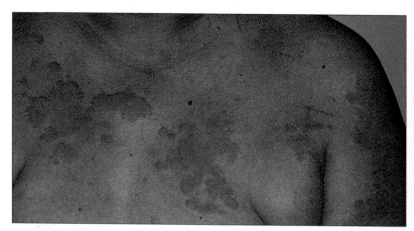

Figure 648. Urticaria. Urticaria is an IgE-mediated reaction. The diet, over-the-counter products, recent illnesses and medication history should be reviewed for any new potential allergens. If the condition becomes chronic (> 6 weeks), laboratory work-up may be performed. (See also **Figure 109.**)

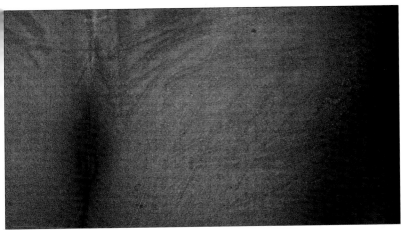

Figure 649. Dermatographism. The patient with dermatographism may present with the chief complaint of itching. Only rarely will he/she say, "My skin turns red and becomes raised wherever I scratch it", although this is exactly what occurs, and is illustrated here. Dermatographism may occur in various clinical situations, including the third trimester of pregnancy or after treatment for scabies. The diagnosis may be established by taking a tongue blade and stroking it several times across the back. Immediate redness will occur in most people but true whealing will develop within minutes in patients with dermatographism.

Figure 650. Cholinergic urticaria. 1–4 mm urticarial papules that occur within minutes of exercise are characteristic. The patient can be made to exercise to the point of sweating in the office or just outside to establish the diagnosis.

335

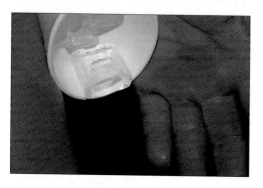

Figure 651. Cold urticaria. Urticarial lesions develop on the fingers after exposure to the cold. Fullness of the throat or swelling of the lips may occur when drinking cold liquids or eating ice cream. Swelling of the head, face and ears may occur after coming indoors from the cold. The ice-cube test is performed as follows: apply two ice cubes to the forearm for 10 minutes. Watch for whealing minutes after removal.

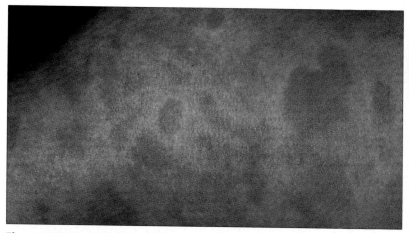

Figure 652. Urticarial vasculitis. Urticarial lesions that last more than 24 hours in any given spot are characteristic. After the initial lesion resolves, purpura remains, as illustrated here. In the acute stage, diascopy will blanch the erythema, allowing visualization of the purpura. Histology shows a leukocytoclastic vasculitis. Urticarial vasculitis is not a specific disease but instead a clinical finding that is usually associated with a vasculitis that causes significant permeability of the dermal microvascular. Diseases that have been associated or have similar lesions include lupus erythematosus, viral hepatitis, cryoglobulins and Schnitzler's syndrome. (See also **Figure 111**.)

For related disease, see also solar urticaria (**Figure 439**.)

Vascular Lesions

Figure 653. Facial telangiectasias, face. Telangiectasias are small blood vessels that may be seen running just below the surface of the skin. They commonly develop on the face of people as they age.

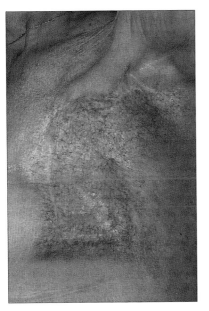

Figure 654. Chronic radiation dermatitis, multiple telangiectasias. Years after radiation exposure, the skin becomes indurated and atrophic with mottled pigmentation and telangiectasias. This woman's breast cancer radiation port has developed such changes.

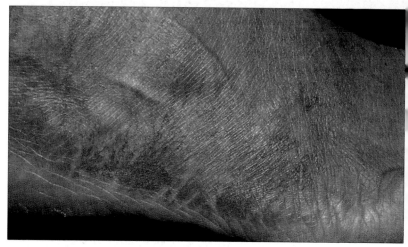

Figure 655. Generalized essential telangiectasia. Benign cutaneous telangiectasias that may involve any part of the skin occur in generalized essential telangiectasia. No systemic bleeding is associated.

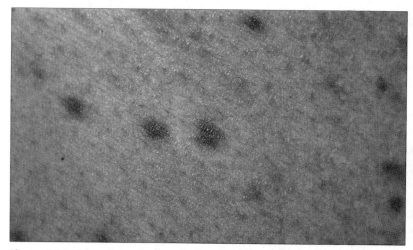

Figure 656. Telangiectasia macularis eruptiva perstans. This variant of mastocytosis presents with telangiectatic macules, often on the trunk of a woman. Special stains (e.g. Giemsa) may be needed to help identify the mast cells histologically. (See also **Figures 22 and 98–100**.)

Figure 657. Spider angiomas. An arcade of vessels radiating out from a central arteriole results in the characteristic appearance. Compressing the central point blanches the arcade. It is very common in children, in pregnancy and with liver disease. (See also **Figure 87**.)

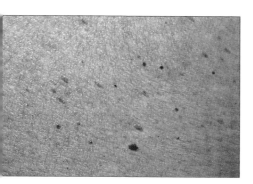

Figure 658. Cherry hemangiomas. Most adults over 30 have one or more red, vascular papules on the trunk. Sometimes, they appear almost 'petechial' as 1–2 mm red macules. In one study of adults 30–39 years of age, 90% of the men and 65% of the women had at least one cherry angioma.

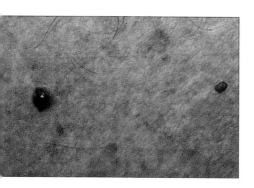

Figure 659. Cherry hemangiomas. The lesion on the right is a true 'cherry' angioma because of its color. The lesion on the left is dark blue because it contains relatively deoxygenated blood.

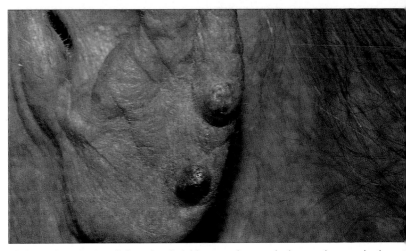

Figure 660. Venous lake. This dark blue vascular papule that can be completely compressed is common on the lips, ears and face.

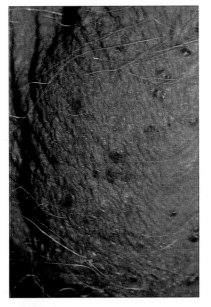

Figure 661. Angiokeratomas, scrotum. Small, 1–6 mm vascular, red papules on the scrotum of an older man are characteristic. They are benign and are usually found incidentally.

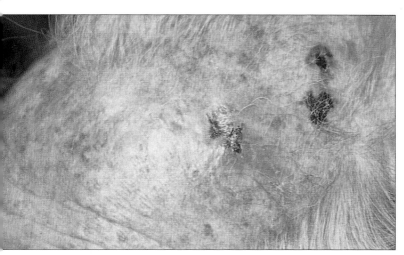

Figure 662. Angiosarcoma of the head and neck. A bruise-like lesion of the head or neck in an elderly patient is characteristic. Vascular papules, nodules or plaques, ulceration and bleeding are common. This highly aggressive vascular tumor may lead to death from local invasion or distant metastases. (Courtesy of Duane Whitaker, MD.)

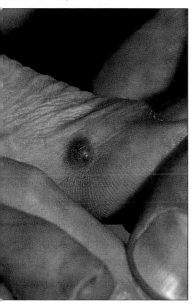

Figure 663. Kaposi's sarcoma, classic type. A reddish-blue to purple papulonodule or plaque beginning on the toe or sole in a man of Southern or Eastern European descent is characteristic. Slow progression may occur with lesions ascending the leg to all parts of the body. Many other organs may be involved but because of the slow progression of the disease, most patients die of unrelated causes.

For related diseases, see also hereditary hemorrhagic telangiectasia (**Figure 73**) and angiokeratoma, thrombosed (**Figure 448**.)

Vasculopathies

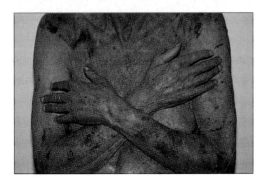

Figure 664. Purpura secondary to topical steroids. Chronic use of topical corticosteroids can result in thinning of the skin, purpura and stretch marks. This older patient had used clobetasol propionate for several months to control his subacute cutaneous lupus erythematosus.

Figure 665. Progressive pigmentary dermatosis. The sudden appearance on the lower legs of many bright red petechiae is characteristic. Some have likened the appearance to Cayenne pepper. Later, the lesions turn brown. The underlying process is a capillaritis, resulting in extravasation of blood. Most often, no cause is known, although certain drugs or vitamins may be implicated.

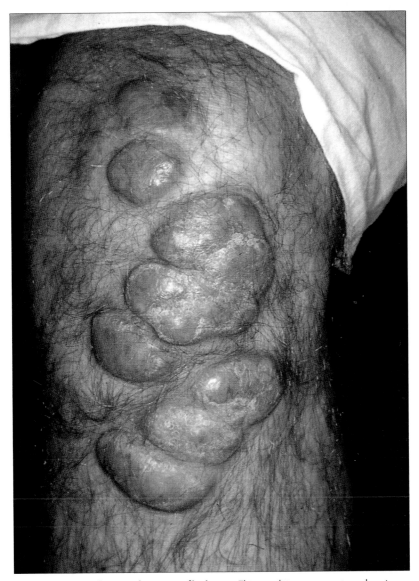

Figure 666. Erythema elevatum diutinum. This condition represents a chronic leukocytoclastic vasculitis. Red–brown nodules are found symmetrically on the dorsa of the hands, elbows and knees. (Courtesy of Gary Cole, MD.)

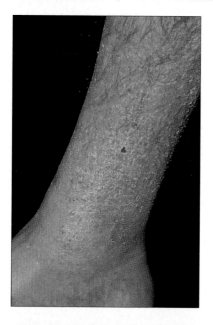

Figure 667. Stasis dermatitis. A red, scaly rash over the medial part of the ankle associated with pitting edema in an older, often overweight, individual is characteristic. The entire lower leg may be involved. Severe edema may lead to beads of fluid and bulla formation. In later stages, the skin may develop a red–brown hue secondary to hemosiderin deposition. Allergic contact dermatitis to topical medication may complicate the clinical picture.

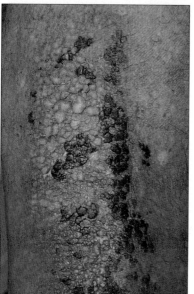

Figure 668. Elephantiasis verruciformis nostra. A chronically enlarged, edematous leg or legs with a verrucous or cobble-stoned surface is characteristic. Stemmer's sign (thickening of the skin over the dorsal toes or fingers) is an early change. Recurrent cellulitis is a frequent finding. The disease results from blockage of the lymphatics (e.g. by venous stasis, malignancy). Elephantiasis of the legs, scrotum, penis and vulva may occur in some parts of the world from lymphatic obstruction by filaria.

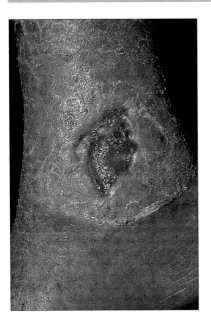

Figure 669. Venous ulcer. Venous ulceration may occur in the setting of chronic stasis. An X-ray to rule out osteomyelitis or a biopsy to rule out malignancy may be indicated for prolonged ulcers. Osteoarthritis, stroke, rheumatoid arthritis or obesity are common contributory factors.

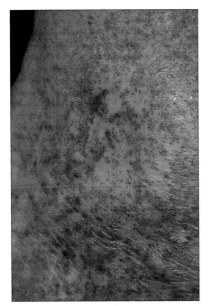

Figure 670. Atrophie blanche. Smooth, white, stellate plaques about the ankle and foot in a woman with chronic venous insufficiency are characteristic of atrophie blanche. The initial lesion is often a purpuric papule or a hemorrhagic bulla followed by a painful ulcer. The stellate, white scar results on healing.

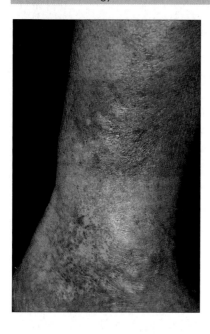

Figure 671. Lipodermatosclerosis.
Also known as sclerosing panniculitis, lipodermatosclerosis manifests itself as an indurated, adherent, erythematous well-defined area on the medial aspect of the lower leg in the setting of chronic venous insufficiency. The lesion may be elevated, flat or depressed. A biopsy should be avoided if possible as healing will invariably be difficult. In this figure, the red plaque represents lipodermato-sclerosis. Ankle flare and atrophie blanche are seen on the medial ankle.

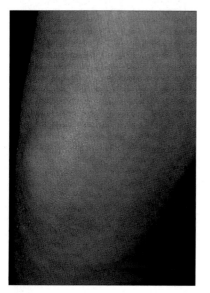

Figure 672. Cutis marmorata.
A reticulated or mottled appearance of the skin in response to cold is characteristic. It is common in infants but may affect all ages.

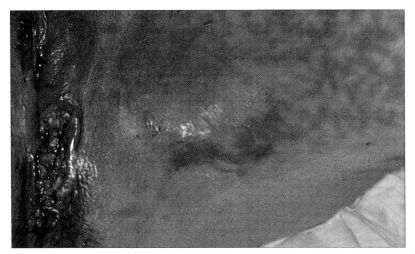

Figure 673. Erythema ab igne. A reticulated pattern of erythema and later hyperpigmentation at the site of chronic thermal exposure (e.g. from a heater, heating pad, fire) is characteristic. The thermal damage preferentially occurs in the border areas between the blood-dispersing arterial zones because the heat dispersion in these areas is low. This 41-year-old woman also has a squamous cell carcinoma arising from the anus. (Courtesy of Paul Koonings, MD.)

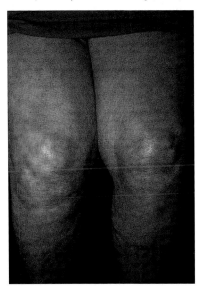

Figure 674. Livedo reticularis. A reticulated, blanching, vascular pattern of the legs occurs as a cutaneous sign of underlying vascular obstructive disease in livedo reticularis. The general work-up should include taking a history (recent infection, drug ingestion, history of cerebrovascular accident or hypertension), a biopsy deep enough to sample medium and large arteries, antinuclear antibody, rheumatoid factor, erythrocyte sedimentation rate, anticardiolipin antibody (positive in this case), antineutrophil cytoplasmic antibody, cryoglobulins, complete blood count and renal and hepatic blood tests.

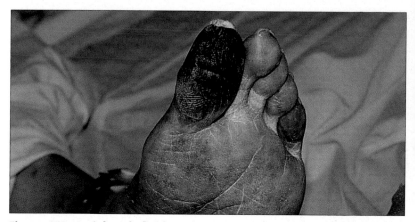

Figure 675. Antiphospholipid syndrome, necrotic toe. Widespread dusky erythema, cutaneous necrosis, leg ulceration, livedo reticularis, splinter hemorrhages and ecchymosis all occur in the antiphospholipid syndrome. The diagnosis requires that a patient has recurrent thrombosis (e.g. deep vein thrombosis, pulmonary emboli, cerebral infarction) or fetal loss (e.g. abortion, intrauterine death) and a positive antiphospholipid antibody. The disease may be primary or secondary (occurring in association with other diseases, the classic being systemic lupus erythematosus) or as a familial trait.

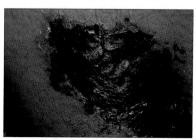

Figure 676. Coumadin necrosis.
Necrosis of the skin 3–6 days after starting warfarin or 3–6 days after excessive hypocoagulability in a patient on warfarin is characteristic. The skin is initially painful and edematous, followed by ecchymosis, hemorrhagic bulla and necrosis. The presumed mechanism is via the more rapid initial decrease in the protein C anticoagulant activity compared with the slower decline of other vitamin K-dependant factors.

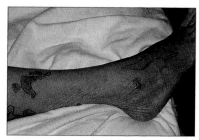

Figure 677. Disseminated intravascular coagulation.
Widespread areas of necrosis in a patient who is profoundly ill are characteristic. The loss of normal inhibition of clotting mechanisms leads to intravascular coagulation associated with consumption of platelets and clotting factors. Associated/underlying diseases include Gram-negative sepsis and shock. The skin marks seen here help to monitor progression.

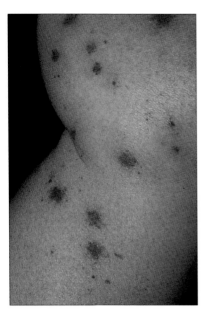

Figure 678. Hypersensitivity vasculitis. Hypersensitivity to a medication can precipitate a cutaneous small vessel vasculitis. Often this is called necrotizing vasculitis or allergic angiitis. (See also **Figure 220**.)

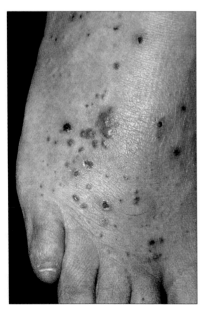

Figure 679. Henoch–Schönlein purpura, adult. Henoch–Schönlein purpura may occur in adults. When the skin is involved, it may present with palpable purpura, as shown here. The pathogenesis involves deposition of immune complexes in which most of the antibody is of the IgA class. A variety of target antigens may be involved (e.g. infectious agents). (See also **Figure 117**.)

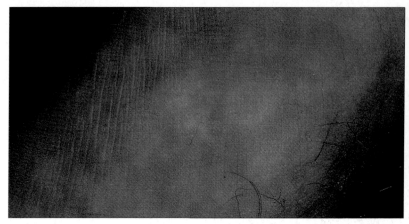

Figure 680. Polyarteritis nodosa. The small and medium-sized arteries are affected by a necrotizing vasculitis which leads to palpable purpura, punched out ulcers, tender subcutaneous nodules and livedo reticularis (shown here). Fever, malaise, myalgias, arthralgias, arthritis, cardiac insufficiency, renal aneurysms and polyneuropathy may occur. A related and possibly causative antigen should be sought, e.g. hepatitis B, HIV and, in children, recent streptococcal infection. (Courtesy of James Rasmussen, MD.)

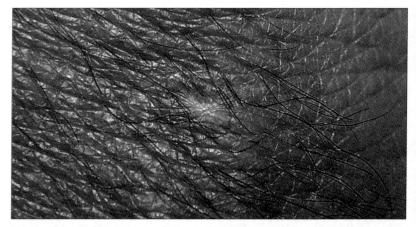

Figure 681. Malignant atrophic papulosis (Dego's disease). Erythematous papules on the trunk and proximal extremities that develop into atrophic, white, porcelain-centered lesions in a young to middle aged man are characteristic. A wedge-shaped area of necrosis is seen histologically in this disease, also known as Dego's disease. The gastrointestinal tract is the second most commonly involved organ, especially the small intestine.

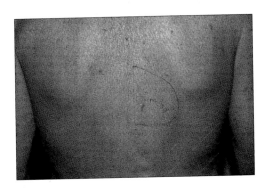

Figure 682. Notalgia paresthetica. Middle-aged to elderly patients may present with a very pruritic, fixed spot on the back just to one side of the midline. Notalgia paresthetica is thought to represent a sensory neuropathy, as the cutaneous nerves take a right angle in their course to innervate that location. Hyperpigmentation may be present and in most patients is thought to be secondary to chronic scratching.

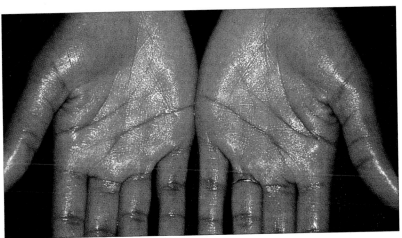

Figure 683. Hyperhidrosis. Excessive sweating of the axilla, palms and soles occurs in hyperhidrosis. For some reason, patients often do not believe there is treatment for this disease and thus do not seek medical attention. The doctor may notice the condition when shaking hands with the patient who is being seen for another reason. Often patients will carry around a tissue or paper towel and dry their hands just before shaking.

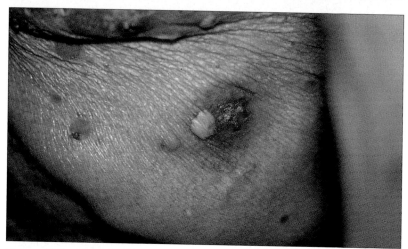

Figure 684. Subcorneal pustular dermatosis. In this chronic pustular dermatosis, also known as Sneddon–Wilkinson disease, sterile superficial pustules develop with a preference for the trunk, axillae and the flexor aspect of the limbs. Annular lesions occur. A direct immunofluorescence should be obtained (and found negative) to exclude intraepidermal neutrophilic IgA dermatosis. (Courtesy of Gary Cole, MD.)

Index